MORALS AND MEDICINE

Discussions from the BBC Third programme

MORALS AND MEDICINE

British Broadcasting Corporation

Published by the
British Broadcasting Corporation
35 Marylebone Street
London WIM 4AA

SBN 563 08590 8

First published 1970

Printed in England
by Ebenezer Baylis & Son Limited
The Trinity Press, Worcester, and London

CONTENTS

FOREWORD

IN THE autumn of 1968 the Department of Extra-Mural Studies in the University of Liverpool announced that they proposed to organise six discussion meetings on 'Morals and Medicine' covering such emotive topics as experiments on human beings, contraception, abortion, and so on. I explored with the Director, Professor Tom Kelly, the possibility of the BBC recording these discussions, in the hope that they might yield broadcasts for the Third Programme, and received his full support.

When the discussions took place, both Professor Kelly's hopes and mine were realised in full measure: his in that there were virtual traffic-jams outside the University on the evenings of the discussions so many people wanted to attend; and mine in that a series of valuable broadcasts resulted. These were broadcast early in 1969 and repeated in midsummer.

Each session consisted of two papers presenting medical and ethical viewpoints, and these were followed by questions to the speakers. This form was retained in the broadcasts but dictates of programme time necessitated vigorous cutting and the elimination of topics of purely Liverpudlian significance.

What is published here is as much of the papers and discussions as could be deemed to be of universal interest, with the exception of the paper by Professor A. Phillips Griffiths, who after careful consideration decided against the publication of his material.

One other point must be emphasised. The figures quoted by Professor T. N. A. Jeffcoate in relation to abortions and the working of the Abortion Act are those given by him at the time. They have not been up-dated. Shortly before going to press, however, the following statistics were given in Hansard for 9 March 1970. In answer to a question from Sir G. Nabarro, the Secretary of State for Social Services stated that in England and Wales during 1969 about 62 per cent of all notified abortions had been carried out in NHS hospitals and 38 per cent in approved places. Ten per cent of the notifications were in respect of women normally resident outside the United Kingdom and these operations were practically all carried out in the approved places. There were 15 deaths attributed to abortion. As Professor Jeffcoate says in his paper, before the passing of the 1967 Act the number of deaths resulting from illegal abortions is not accurately known but it is quoted as having been in the region of 50 per annum.

The proceedings throughout were conducted by the President of the General Medical Council, Lord Cohen of Birkenhead, whose valuable interventions on points of medical ethics have been retained, although, in the interests of space, his formal remarks have had to go.

As editor of the radio programmes and now of these extended versions I wish to thank both Lord Cohen and Professor Tom Kelly for their help in organising six outstanding contributions to the dialogue of our time.

ARCHIE CLOW

I KEEPING PEOPLE ALIVE

HENRY MILLER & ANTHONY BLOOM

MILLER My approach to this problem is based on a philosophical viewpoint that is, to my mind, none the worse for being currently unfashionable. To me the history of man is the history of his increasing understanding and control of the physical world and of an unremitting struggle to maintain supremacy over his biological competitors. With this has come a decline in the influence of religions and other superstitions and an increasing conviction that attempts to improve the here-and-now should take precedence over the search for consolation in a hypothetical thereafter. In this view our energies are better directed to pursuing what Sir Peter Medawar has epitomised as 'the art of the soluble' than to fruitless speculation about the unknowable.

The present unpopularity of such an orientation is due, in part, to the very success of the scientific method in the mastery of our environment. It is easy for the fearful to maintain that the gains we owe to the scientific revolution are insubstantial and are outweighed by the perils inherent in the failure of political competence to keep abreast of scientific achievement. For the present, our ability to understand and manipulate the physical world has clearly outrun our capacity to devise an appropriate social framework for the effective application of new knowledge and new skills. It is tempting to wonder whether some of our problems might be met by replacing unsuccessful statesmen with successful scientists. But the honest materialist must admit to his suspicion that the difficulties of the politician and the triumphs of the scientist reflect the relative intractabilities of their materials rather than the respective skill of the operators.

However, most of our present difficulties are at any rate man-made, remediable, and probably transient, while our gains are enormous and permanent. In one field of medicine that is under discussion in this chapter we need look no further than the conquest of bacterial infection, which has already relieved more human suffering than has been caused by all the wars of the present century. For despite its actual and hypothetical dangers to mankind, the advance of science has already improved the quality of life for millions of the world's inhabitants. Although scientific materialism is an unfashionable philosophy, and an optimistic materialism even more out of tune with the cultivated pessimism that is so popular today, it is, in fact, the philosophical basis on which most of us organise our lives, whatever creed we profess.

At this stage the reader may reasonably object that the moral neutralism of the scientific attitude precludes its relevance to our discussion. My reply is simple. The reason for a moral code is pragmatic and arises in the first instance from our need to live together without killing one another and at a more advanced stage of sophistication to desist from making life too uncomfortable for one another. The scientist's approach to morals is utilitarian. The fact that it quite often happens to coincide with the attitudes of Christianity indicates that even the most improbable of religions has to keep its feet on the ground if it is to remain relevant. The utilitarian opposes slaughtering people because he is concerned that others should have no excuse for slaughtering him. This is the basis of law, which is the very essence of human civilisation. And although the condition of the world today furnishes many arguments for pessimism in the short term, it is worth remembering that some kind of law obtains today over a wider area of the earth's surface than at any time in history.

Medicine has changed more radically in the past thirty years than in the previous two centuries. Science has endowed us with remarkable opportunities for changing the course of serious illness just as it has transformed our lives in many other ways. Thirty years ago the role of medicine was mostly consolatory. Today there are some diseases like syphilis that can be rapidly cured, others like poliomyelitis that can be prevented, many like kidney disease that can be greatly relieved – all by treatments that were unheard of a quarter of a century ago. Such developments have relieved physicians of some anxiety but the freedom of choice that they imply has posed new responsibilities. Some new forms of treatment are complicated and harrowing for the patient as well as expensive to society. There are undoubtedly instances where it is kinder to withhold them than to prolong a painful and miserable existence by their employment.

Such decisions are often difficult, but experience suggests that little would be gained from shifting the responsibility from the physician in charge of the patient to a committee, however impeccable and well-intentioned. The physician is trained to take such decisions, he alone is in possession of the full facts of the illness and is better equipped to weigh its imponderables than anyone else. He knows the possibilities, the risks and the discomforts attendant on complex treatment, and he is able to decide what he would like done if he himself were the patient. This is, emphatically, the final basis of decision in such dilemmas.

In the past the issue to treat or not to treat was often determined by the patient's social status and his ability to afford the methods then in vogue. In the past also, ironically, the patient unable to afford treatment was often spared ordeals that were ineffective, gruelling, and frankly harmful to his chances of survival. Today the pervasiveness of mass communication and the popularity of medical radio and television programmes have brought the doctor's dilemmas into every living-room. Most of the population of Great Britain know that a large number of young and otherwise healthy lives could be saved by making artificial kidney treatment generally available. And those with any knowledge of the matter know that this is not being done very quickly. It is fashionable to regret television publicity for medical matters, but it is important that the public should be informed of what modern medicine has to offer, so that in the end even politicians may come to accord the preservation of life and health a higher priority than preparations for its destruction.

The problems that face the doctors of today in connection with keeping people alive can be exemplified by some actual clinical situations. Motives are always mixed, and shortage of nursing staff was undoubtedly one reason for the development of intensive treatment – the aim being to concentrate nursing and other technical skills where they were most needed, rather than to spread them thinly over many parts of the hospital's widely differing needs. The development of new methods of recording the patient's progress, such as continuous automatic recordings of cardiac activity, and the ability to maintain artificial respiration almost indefinitely as well as repeatedly to restart the patient's heart after its arrest by disease, also contributed to the development of intensive care. At the present time a combination of public and professional pressure is leading to the establishment of such units in most of our major hospitals. As often happens, economies in one direction, in nursing, have been outweighed by the increasing cost of new and more sophisticated techniques. And since these costs must be met from hospital revenues that are always well below that considered necessary by the responsible hospital authority, difficult questions of priority at the local level are inescapable. Nor is it easy to compare the results of treatment in the intensive care unit with those obtained by simpler methods. Work in such units is harrowing and exacting and, for the most part, they are in the hands of dedicated enthusiasts convinced, probably rightly, of the effectiveness of their methods. Unfortunately the enthusiastic innovator is rarely an objective assessor and is inclined to neglect the phase of carefully controlled trial that should always precede the general adoption of any new technique as a routine procedure. Once the method is thus established, anything in the nature of objective trial becomes doubly difficult. We still lack, for example, the basic data that could permit a valid comparison of the outlook for coronary thrombosis treated with all the paraphernalia of a modern cardiac unit with that of an identical patient who takes his chance at home with morphia, whisky and commercial television. And the cautious physician cannot but recall the uncritical enthusiasm that recently threatened to put an appreciable proportion of the adult population on long-term anticoagulant drugs. That some patients whose hearts are no longer beating can be resuscitated by an electric shock is beyond doubt, but the contribution to survival rate implicit in this fact is only one amongst many variables that may affect the critical question of the patient's survival under intensive treatment or without it in his own home.

However, there are many instances in which intensive treatment certainly saves life. One example is the terrifying failure of respiration that occurs in certain acute and entirely recoverable diseases in the nervous system. Another is severe head injury, where the maintenance of physiological function and biochemical balance during prolonged unconsciousness may make all the difference between death and recovery. Many patients with severe head injury, who would otherwise certainly have died, survive in a modern neurosurgical unit. And although a very occasional case may be mentally or physically crippled, the large majority not only survive but return to work. In the acute stage of head injury prediction is impossible, and all must be given the chance of survival. In most patients resuscitation is unnecessary. In a few, evidence of cerebral damage is so gross that attempts can be discounted. But there are many others in whom the outlook may remain uncertain for days or even longer. Many of these are otherwise healthy young people injured in traffic accidents, and most of us would give a very high priority to making expert intensive treatment available to all such cases for as long as there is the faintest hope of recovery.

Intensive treatment is sometimes misused. It is unkind to submit the very elderly or chronically decrepit to what is undoubtedly a harrowing experience and, like most physicians, I have had doctors as patients who specifically requested that they should be spared the ordeal. On the other hand we owe it to the patient when the outcome is in doubt. Quite often it buys time for definitive diagnosis so that we can more accurately predict the ultimate outcome. In other instances we persist to the end where a desperately severe disease is theoretically recoverable. But the decision to submit a patient to resuscitation or intensive therapy must be informed and deliberate and taken at a responsible level. When damage is clearly irrevocable and irrecoverable the physician must steel himself not to prolong life artificially beyond the point at which the patient's interests are served. If expert investigation of a head-injured patient reveals damage to the brain so gross that it precludes survival the doctor must overcome his reluctance to disconnect the respirator, so that scarce resources are not denied to others who might have been saved.

Kidney disease kills the affected patient because the diseased organs fail to clear the blood of poisonous chemical substances produced in the course of metabolism. The idea of leading the patient's blood from an artery to an artificial filter outside the body and passing it back into a vein is ingeniously simple, though its development as a practical technique was anything but easy. Kidney damage sometimes occurs acutely as a result of chemical poisoning, or changes induced by severe general injury, and the use of the artificial kidney preserves life during the period of days which give the patient's kidneys time to recover. However, it soon became clear that dialysis – the artificial kidney – was also effective in patients with progressive deterioration of kidney function occurring as a terminal event in chronic disease. The fact that many of these chronic cases can be relieved and maintained in tolerable health by the use of the artificial kidney over a period of years gives the problem of keeping people alive a particular relevance at the present time. About seven thousand people die each year in Britain from chronic kidney disease. And of these probably about two thousand could probably be saved by long-term dialysis if it were generally available. To treat all those who could benefit would cost about thirty million pounds a year and would employ about ten thousand trained personnel. Thirty million pounds a year sounds a lot of money but it is in fact less than half of what we already spend on the care of the mentally defective. This is not a question of equipment, but of people trained and willing to undertake work that is exacting, skilful and tedious. Progress in the direction of furnishing these facilities is slow. Government can plead with some reason that quite apart from money the people are just not available to do the job. It is wrong to be patient with a system of social priorities that does not give the saving of life the very highest priority. There was a time when similar decisions had to be made about the use of scanty supplies of penicillin. We need firmer reassurance than we have so far received that the organisation of a service for dialysis is being given the same kind of priority that production of penicillin was given in the 1940s. It is even more important that we train and organise a medical profession equipped in total and individual capacity to avert similar tragic delays in the application of other new methods of treatment already coming into view.

Euthanasia is a much discussed but, to my mind, less important issue. I can see no very strong arguments against its legalisation at the patient's request in hopelessly fatal disease. However, my own experience suggests that such a patient is usually so desperately ill that clouding of consciousness would often jeopardise his competence to decide. I agree with the supporters of euthanasia that the physician's main duty is to relieve pain and to sustain and improve the quality of life by relief of suffering, rather than primarily to prolong it. But in my experience there are few fatal illnesses in which the last weeks or months cannot be made tolerable by the generous use of drugs. I know there are exceptions, such as the occasional patients who are clearly conscious, but humiliated by the progressive rotting of their bodies from such destructive disease as gynaecological cancer, without hope of recovery, and distressed by being a burden to others as well as to themselves. In such a case the surgeon who eases the patient's end by an intravenous injection of morphia is acting in the best traditions of his profession. But this is a most exceptional situation between doctor and patient and one that is unlikely to be affected one way or the other by legislation.

Development in the speciality of pediatric surgery has focused attention on the treatment of the infant born with a congenital defect. In this field there have been therapeutic triumphs where the relief of an isolated anomaly produces a healthy infant instead of a dead baby. However, there are other aspects of this sort of surgery that cause grave concern in the medical profession, and which, to my mind, pose more real moral problems than any of those already discussed. A good example is spina bifida, which at the present time is the subject of a great deal of sustained and enthusiastic surgical activity, both in Britain and abroad. There can be no doubt that successful operation in minor cases of this congenital defect in the spinal column saves life by preventing infection. And, in the absence of paralysis, all surgeons would favour operation. In severe cases with paralysis, surgery is a different matter and highly controversial. Some lives could be saved, and some children would survive who would have succumbed without surgical intervention, often during the first year of life. The real problem is, what sort of survival? Surgical enthusiasts can quote remarkable successes, but some children who survive are physically and even mentally crippled, presenting a distressing and formidable responsibility both to their families and to society. One special difficulty in this instance is that the decision as to whether or not to operate has to be made almost immediately after birth. To refer an infant to a surgeon is virtually to request operation. The parents are in no position to deliberate over the indications or contra-indications for surgical treatment, and are torn between a desire that the child should survive at all costs and a gradually dawning comprehension as to the problems of the future. The general practitioner or pediatrician can be guided only by his own feelings, or his own judgement as to what he would wish done if he were the parent of the child. For myself, I do not believe we are under any obligation to take exceptional measures to ensure survival in the presence of any severe congenital abnormality that cannot be genuinely cured by surgery. I think many of my professional colleagues and their wives share this view, and are grateful to the doctor who does not institute elaborate and dramatic measures to ensure survival in the grossly abnormal baby.

My contribution to this discussion is wide open to the criticism that it is pragmatic, that it side-steps the moral issues we are supposed to be considering and, of course, that it is professionally orientated. These criticisms are entirely valid, but my approach *is* professional. The issue of keeping people alive is not a new one. It has been faced by doctors over the ages. The contributions of science to medicine crowd in upon us. They raise problems that are more urgent and more dramatic than in the past, but in essence they are no different. The training of a physician, the whole philosophical outlook of a physician, has been directed to relieving suffering and to maintaining life for as long as it has anything to offer to the patient. To my mind, metaphysical considerations are otiose. I am a professional and, if the matter came to trial, I would trust myself to the empirical enthusiasm of Christian Barnard rather than to the windy metaphysics of Malcolm Muggeridge.

BLOOM I would like to attempt to examine this problem from another angle. The moral problem which is faced by patient and family on one side and by the physician on the other, is given significance by the evaluation of life and of death: according to what we think of life and what we think of death, we are bound to take decisions in different directions. So is it the role of the physician, of the family, or of each of us, to try to survive at all costs, or not? This is the first question. And when I say survive, I mean continue to exist physically and to try to drag this physical existence to the last possible limit.

I was brought up with old-fashioned beliefs, to which I still subscribe. My father used to say that my life has no value or significance beyond what it is devoted to, so the physical presence, or absence, of a person is not to me the decisive feature. A person *has* absolute significance, but not simply because he chanced to come into the world, and throughout his life was useless, parasitic, or evil. There is an evaluation of life which is founded on something else. This is important, because when we have to take decisions as to the life or death of a man in conjunction with the life and death of another, as in the case of transplants, we must have some criterion for judgement. And when I say we, I do not mean only the physician, but the family, the patient and perhaps society. But it is not merely the social utility of a given person that is the decisive feature. A person may appear to have little scope or influence, and yet in the small field in which he lives, acts, works, be very essential.

I think that if we begin by asking ourselves what we stand for in life, whether we wish simply to survive as long as possible, or whether we wish to live for a purpose – to make our lives significant and meaningful – we could perhaps then decide beforehand what we are prepared to endure and what we are prepared to contribute to the life and death of others. Along this line of thought, each of us could make a decision as to whether we are prepared to give our heart, our kidneys or any other part that may, at the time of our death, be needed by another, and carry a card indicating our will or readiness. That would be part of life, not part of death. The laying down of one's life is part of living, and not part of dying in the sense in which so often people think of death – as coming to an end, or enduring final defeat.

Leaving for a moment this question of life and its appraisal, what about death? One of the things that strikes me so often in this country is the way death is pushed aside. To me this speaks of a morbid attitude to death. If we want to face the problem of death and of preserving life and see it as something more than the necessity to keep people alive for as long as they can survive, then we must have a positive, or a different attitude to death. This is something which I believe physicians, as well as others, should face more thoughtfully than they do – think about it, face it, be together with the dying, reflect on it, and have a real, not evasive, attitude to death. Death is always ambiguous. If I were a straight unbeliever, I would have less problems with death, because I should see in it merely a process that belongs to natural history. I could be pained, or hurt, by the fact that someone I love had died, and grieved by separation, but there is no tragedy in that kind of death. It is natural, and nature is good; a fact has no moral connotation if there is no other way of approaching it. But for a believer – and I am speaking from the point of view of a Christian believer – death is ambiguous. On the one hand, it is an evil which we cannot accept because we believe that man was not created to die, and that mortality is an evil in our human condition; and on the other hand, death is the only way in which we can outgrow the limitations of a world that has gone wrong, a world in which, instead of eternity, there can be only evil endlessness. In that respect death has a positive significance. If you do not equate life with your mere physical presence and if you do not equate death with destruction and defeat, if life has meaning because of what it stands for, what it is devoted to, what it is given for, laid down for, then one can face death differently. And in the moral decisions which we must take, with regard to a dying person – including ourselves because we are all prospective corpses – we must remember that we are all afflicted with an incurable disease which is mortality. So I think we must have the courage to look at our lives and say 'our life is no life'. It can become useful only if I lay it down, only if I am prepared to give myself that others may live.

An example can be taken from the expedition of Captain Scott to the Antarctic, when one of his companions, crippled by cold, walked into the storm and died that the others might return. It was an act of supreme life and it was a meeting with death that made sense. Every one of us is not in the Antarctic and cannot walk into the storm, yet every one of us is in a situation in which we either help or impede someone's life or the lives of the people around us. At times, to be prepared to give one's body that others may live is a creative and meaningful act. On the other hand, death is coming towards each of us, and we must be able to face it creatively, and here again, life and death are interwoven. When practical medical decisions are to be taken, what is the basis for them? How can we evaluate a patient's worth? The physician must make a decision which is related to the individual and to nothing else. This person must be helped to live or allowed to die, but both must be positively decided and not simply undergone and endured. The deciding criteria are health or disease, plenitude of life or something that appears as being a lessened life.

At this point I think we must be very careful. I am not thinking now of babies born under conditions that will not allow them to live and to develop, but of people who have undergone, in the course of their lives, accidents, or injuries, that make them, from a cold-blooded and cynical point of view, a burden to society. And this brings me to the problem of euthanasia. I think that we must all submit ourselves to undergo an earnest rethinking about suffering, an earnest training in facing suffering, because my impression is that, very often, people could face suffering which they refuse to face for no other reason than cowardice, and the result of this is that people become less and less capable of facing lesser and lesser suffering. In the end, this policy of escape leads to continuous mental suffering, because when suffering is not there it is expected and feared, and it overshadows life. We should train ourselves knowingly, systematically, to face suffering, both moral and physical, to push back the limits which we so easily assign to the use of drugs for a headache, for a toothache, for the fear of it, for the possibility of it. That way we might begin to give enormous significance to suffering as an act of human fortitude and human greatness, as we can see throughout the ages in a variety of people in all kinds of civilisation.

MILLER I think the Archbishop has demonstrated some differences that are worth discussion. I think the basic difference between materialist and Christian concerns especially this matter of suffering. A materialist regards all suffering as inherently bad, and cheerfully takes his tablet for the toothache. He does not believe that by withholding the tablet, he will in any way ennoble himself. He thinks he will probably be a more unpleasant as well as a more uncomfortable person with the toothache than with the tablet. I do agree that there is a good deal of mock suffering in order to obtain all kinds of ends, and that some of what passes in psychiatric circles for neurosis is not illness at all but an unscrupulous attempt to evade social or personal responsibilities. But in the case of euthanasia we are discussing real suffering in very grave illness. I have no enthusiasm for euthanasia, but I think there are times when something closely approaching euthanasia is imperative. In general, however, I think that suffering is more inclined to distort than to ennoble the personality.

I don't think there are many other serious differences of opinion between myself and Dr Bloom. I quite agree that we do not want to survive at all costs. On the other hand, I think the Archbishop's discussion of the purpose of survival takes me into an area about which I cannot pretend even to guess. It seems to me that so long as life is, in balance, more pleasant than unpleasant, one would want to survive. If the pain or the distress were irremediable, one would probably not wish to survive. This is so in theory, but indeed in practice very few people except for the mentally ill wish not to survive, however desperate their predicament, and this is one reason why I believe that voluntary and deliberate euthanasia would have few takers.

I agree that the English run away from death. Perhaps everybody does. But I am surprised that Christians run away from death. To me death means merely the transformation of a certain amount of fat, carbohydrate and protein into other metabolic products, and that's the end of me. However, I have never observed that, when the time comes, those who look forward to a future life of unmitigated bliss show any greater eagerness to embrace it than those with less sanguine expectations. I think that the behaviour of many people with very severe chronic disability is a tremendous lesson to us not to pay much attention to the numerous discomforts that we all have. People with very grave disabilities, like paraplegia, frequently show incredible fortitude, and certainly no desire to die, despite very great suffering. I don't think it is a good thing that there should be paraplegics to convince us of this, but I think they teach us a salutary lesson.

BLOOM If I may just comment on what you have said; I do not think that suffering automatically ennobles anyone. I think it is our attitude to suffering which makes a very important difference to what we are. There are people who are broken by suffering, and this is why I believe that we should submit ourselves and train generation after generation into another attitude different from that of the hare before the dog.

Now to the question of people wanting to die or wanting simply to resign from life. As long as there is something to fight against, people are prepared to fight. But there can be a moment which is very difficult. It is aimless happiness, when happiness seems not to be worth living for. Usually fighting is always worth living for, because we *are* combative. Even when our suffering reaches an incredible degree it is still worth facing. For a year and a half I was a physician in charge of survivors from German concentration camps. I was impressed by the extent of their bravery and their desire to fight. They did not resign, otherwise they would have died by the thousand long before. So when I said that we must have an aim or a content to life, I did not mean simply a metaphysical world outlook but something to strive for that is greater than simple survival and simple plodding along. The people who survive in war are people who want to go back to something. The people who survive in life are the people who live for something and towards something. It is not pie in the sky that allows someone not to be afraid of death. It is the sense of being alive with the quality, depth, and intensity of life which physical disruption cannot impair.

One of the men who impressed me most in my life said to me when I was still a teenager, 'Remember one must wait for death as a young man waits for his girlfriend.' He was not a romantic, and he was not morbid. He lived intensely and expected death as a door that opens with certainty into more life. These are the only people who can face death without fear.

Members of the audience were then invited by the Chairman, Lord Cohen, to put questions to the two speakers.

N. S. BARNETT Professor Miller – you spoke of disconnecting a respirator from a dying patient in order that it might be used on some other patient whose life might thereby be saved. But supposing there were no other patients in existence, what would your attitude be then to disconnecting the respirator?

MILLER I accept your implied criticism of my comment on that, and I would say that one should learn to turn a respirator off anyway if it is no longer helping the patient, irrespective of the question of availability of resources.

BARNETT I should like to ask the Archbishop a question too. Leaving aside the attitude of a person to his own suffering or death, what is your opinion on the right of another person to terminate the sufferer's life?

BLOOM I don't think anyone has the right to terminate someone's life by, say, putting him to sleep, the way we do with cats, but I do believe that a person has the right to allow a relative to die peacefully without being submitted for weeks or months to all the torments one can inflict on a patient in order to make him live longer. If the patient is conscious and can decide with those caring for him, I think it is perfectly legitimate to do nothing and allow him to die a natural death peacefully; a death, that is, which is not artificially postponed. If a person is unconscious, I think one has a right to allow the person to die his natural death, if we know that he is incurable. This has nothing to do with our believing or not believing that this person can survive longer or not – this is not in our hands – but I believe that we have the right not to prolong life indefinitely.

J. HEYES I have a question for Professor Miller. In view of the shortage of equipment for kidney dialysis, I would be interested, as a social worker, to know what terms of reference he uses in considering to which patients he ought to give priority.

MILLER Could I just correct one thing. It is not the shortage of equipment! An artificial kidney machine is not very expensive. It is the problem of personnel to run a very difficult strenuous service. We haven't got the people. I don't run a Kidney Unit but I know people who do, and of course the main criterion is to choose the patient most certain to benefit, just as if one were choosing a patient for any kind of surgical operation. Beyond that I think they try to take into account all kind of ponderables and imponderables including age, family responsibilities; and those difficult social and moral questions on which the Archbishop is a much greater authority than I.

LORD COHEN I wonder if I might put a question which relates to priorities. You said, Professor Miller, that we could keep our 30,000 renal patients alive if we had another 10,000 medical personnel. But is it not true that men and money and management and the resources thereof are limited in this country? Take men, for example. If we had another 10,000 doctors, would that deplete the number of teachers, or engineers and so forth, which we have? Must we not consider education, housing and the like, in all these considerations, and come to some judgement based on priorities?

MILLER I agree, and it is unfortunate that Parliamentary democracy affords few opportunities for serious discussion of priorities. Even in those three weeks before a General Election, where we are presented with the appetising choice of Box or Cox for the next five years, these issues are rarely raised, most of the time being devoted to pointing out the failings of the other party. These priorities are of vital importance, but not easy to determine. Everybody with a vested interest, whether it is in education, housing, or medicine, presses his own case as vigorously as possible. Of the 10,000 people needed for an adequate dialysis service few are doctors, but they are people in at least as short supply, such as first-class technicians and skilled and devoted nurses. What you say is perfectly true, but I think that it is often used to excuse not making every possible effort to train more people. We are not yet scraping the bottom of the barrel of trainable people.

COHEN Could I ask about the example that you chose of the child paralysed with spina bifida, whom you say should not have pediatric surgery. You rather praised the paraplegic, and the tetraplegic, who had shown how they had overcome their disabilities. Supposing you have a child born physically apparently well, but virtually an ament. I am sure you would say that child must remain alive; so you would differentiate, as it were, between the omission of means of saving life, and the commission of means of destroying life. Am I right in that?

MILLER Yes. In other words, I don't think there's any point in operating on a congenital heart defect in a Mongolian idiot, on the other hand there is no excuse for going round slaughtering healthy Mongols.

COHEN I think this really comes down, doesn't it, to A. H. Clough's observation, 'Thou shalt not kill, but needs not strive officiously to keep alive.' I think most doctors would follow that doctrine, don't you?

MILLER Yes.

A. V. NEWTON If I could get back to the issue of the concentration camp, which was raised by the Archbishop. I remember reading a psychiatric report by some doctors, who had examined the inmates of some concentration camps, who were European businessmen. Prior to their entry into the camp they had all suffered from either gastric or duodenal ulcers. Those which survived their stay apparently came through actually free from these particular medical defects, but later on they returned to business life and regained their ulcers. If this particular investigation has any relevance to the real suffering in human existence, would either of the speakers like to comment upon it?

MILLER I am reminded of a remark by a great American teacher of mine, who sat back and listened attentively while a controversial paper was read and whose only comment was 'Interesting, if true . . .'

BLOOM I wouldn't like to be light-minded and draw conclusions which are almost offensive and impertinent. But it impresses me that people who are confronted with the real issues very often grow in stature and can meet them without nervous disease, without mental trouble and without ulcers, while those confronted with things which are too small for human stature, and yet too big for their little standing in life, may develop a lot of trouble, gastric or other. Now, I wouldn't go beyond this and suggest that concentration camps are the best cure for ulcers.

H. H. FRANCIS I would welcome the comments and advice of both speakers on a problem which troubles obstetricians. It is that of performing, or not performing, post-morten Caesarean sections, when the child is at term, presumably normal and definitely alive, and when some catastrophe had suddenly struck down the mother. It is a situation where time is limited. The child will die from asphyxia within ten or fifteen minutes, so that one really has to have decided on a policy in advance, when one reaches a certain stage of responsibility in Obstetrics. I have had to face this problem twice.

It brings in this matter of the consciousness of the foetus, because our brains are all afferent machines, and we need afferent stimuli in order to give us consciousness. The foetus is protected from almost all stimuli, apart from perhaps a few acoustic ones, and so it is in the ordinary sense unconscious. On the first occasion I was faced with this problem, I did proceed to incise the abdomen and the uterus, and produced the child, which was immediately and thereafter completely rejected by the father. He felt that this child had been the cause of his wife's death. And I took the trouble to track down two other successful post-mortem Caesarean sections done in this city and both of those children suffered the same thing. They were given out for adoption, they were utterly rejected, so that on the second occasion, when I was faced with this problem, I decided that perhaps it was better to let the child die with the mother. But I would very much like to hear your views on this particular problem.

MILLER I think this is really extremely difficult, and I would not pretend that I can give an answer to it at all. One tends to be platitudinous and say it depends on the circumstances, but I am aware that is not a good answer. If you had experience in three cases in which it went wrong, there is obviously a case of a sort for doing nothing. But this really is a doctor's dilemma; perhaps an insoluble one. I'd be interested to know what the Archbishop has to say.

BLOOM I don't think you can, simply on the assumption that the family or social life of the child may be different from what you hope it will be, allow the child to die. I think any child which can live, should be allowed to live. You cannot presume to know what will happen next. I dare say that among the millions of children who are born of live mothers into so-called normal families, there are great miseries, and many have to face, if not the hatred of their father, problems that are not less, judging by what one finds in psychiatric clinics, for instance, for children. But I don't think one can take that into account. I think what one can do is to bring the child into the world and, if this is the case, instead of submitting him to the ordeal of having a father who hates him, take intelligent creative steps to give him as normal a life as he can, keeping track of the father, because he may also come to his senses after a shorter, or longer, period of – well, parental insanity.

COHEN Isn't the answer to your question an analogous question? What would you do when a mother, who has actually given birth to a live child, dies during the course of giving birth to the child? Would you leave the child to die? I think the answer is 'No', and I think this is the answer when a child is viable in the womb, whatever be the ultimate social responsibilities and difficulties, and fortunately they are not always as bad as your experience suggests. Some fathers are delighted to have the child who reminds them of their mother, who was part of the mother, who is part of the father. Some of these cases are quite well known and I think, as I say, that the analogous question does answer your question, and that it is only psychological and social circumstances that surround the problem.

D. L. SCOTT I'm asking a question of Professor Miller. As he knows, our intensive care wards are generally working to capacity and often occupied by suicide cases. If such were the situation and a crushed chest road accident came in whose entire survival depended on intensive care, and the only alternative was either to let this patient die or remove the suicide, what would you do under these circumstances?

MILLER Well, the majority of cases of attempted suicide admitted to hospital are suffering from depressive illness, which is treatable and recoverable. Any decision of this kind must be made not on general principles, but must depend on the circumstances of the particular case. The attempted suicide may be a better risk for complete recovery than a very severely physically injured person. And in these circumstances one wouldn't take the attempted suicide off the respirator and put somebody else on it. It seems to me that your question endows suicide with some kind of implied moral obloquy, and suggests that the psychiatric casualty does not really deserve the treatment as much as if he had been careless enough to get run over.

D. R. LEWIN I should like to come back to the question of priorities, this time in the field of medicine only. We are all very impressed by the great work done in kidney transplants and in heart transplants. We are very distressed that several thousand people who could be saved yearly by kidney dialysis are neglected through lack of resources. But I should like to draw attention to a less spectacular activity, but one that could probably have a very much larger impact on the amount of suffering, and the number of deaths in this country; I mean a broad spectrum diagnosis of the general population. There is a little work being done on this, yet it is thought that a large number of illnesses and deaths could be prevented by it. Now this is a question of saving lives, a question of saving one life rather than another, on a very very large magnitude, much larger than deciding to take a respirator from one person to another. Given the present economic stringencies which we are all in, and particularly the NHS, what priority should such screening be given?

MILLER The question argues a rather naïve view, appropriate perhaps to a hospital administrator. The implication is, that the kind of person who goes round knocking on doors and testing people's urine is a man who might otherwise be employed in grafting kidneys. But the two animals are not interchangeable. To tell surgeons that they must stop transplanting organs and get busy dealing with injured hands would be a perfectly legitimate administrative suggestion. But it will merely ensure that those who are already grafting kidneys or doing cardiac transplants will smartly get on the first plane for the United States and we shall never see them again, because they are dedicated pioneers. I would give screening the normal population a very low priority indeed amongst medical investigations. It has been said that the routine medical examination is capable only of detecting pregnancy in its advanced stages! This is a slight exaggeration, but one thing routine screening does is to cause alarm, as anybody knows who has examined people turned down for insurance because of a blood pressure five points above normal. They spend the next three years going to successive cardiologists trying to be persuaded that there is nothing the matter with them. And the other thing, of course, is that screening reveals a whole lot of minor anomalies. Weeks and months of elaborate tests are then needed to prove that they don't mean anything. The expense is not in the initial screening. It is in laying ghosts that would have been better never raised.

FOSTER I would like to hear the two speakers' views on whether they consider the expense and time involved in a heart transplant – in order to keep the patient alive for what, at a maximum, is only a very short time – is justified, in comparison with other uses to which this money and manpower could be put.

BLOOM This is a very technical question and I have been out of medical practice for twenty years now. But from what I know about other kinds of surgery and medical work, most of the operations which are now performed quickly and which give lasting results at a comparatively low cost of effort, at a certain stage took a great deal more time, skill, and so forth. And if we do not start now – doing these operations with great difficulty – there is no reason to imagine that in ten or a hundred years they will be done any better, any quicker, or at any lower cost. But I am not sure that my medical judgement on this point is sound. As to principles, I don't think there are any principles involved here. There is no more principle involved in a heart transplant than in the excision of part of the stomach. There was a time when certain operations were almost beyond doing; now they are not. And I wonder whether heart transplants and others won't soon be in the same position.

MILLER I would agree with everything the Archbishop says. This is perfectly true. I think it unfortunate that cardiac transplantation has received so much publicity. It has done so, of course, because the heart is an interesting organ. It actually beats. It isn't like the kidney which just lies there. On the other hand the same things were being said about kidney transplants five years ago, and yet we now have a method that is not far short of routine in a good surgical hospital. However, in relation to cardiac transplantation I would like to see a little less effort devoted to heroic operation and a little more to the basic research required to develop a reliable procedure.

Cardiac transplantation is jumping the gun before the theoretical basis has been thoroughly prepared. Occasionally it is brilliantly successful, but it is unrealistic at the moment, except on a small and entirely experimental scale.

COHEN In all these fields of ethics it seems to me that there are no rational value judgements. Value judgements depend upon factors other than pure reason. And your attitude towards the problems which present are those which give you the solutions you are looking for. With regard to heart transplants, I believe with Professor Miller that these are courageous attempts by surgeons who feel that they ought not to be delayed. But it was a little jumping the gun and the great trouble has been the unseemly publicity and the sudden chauvinistic attitude of practically every nation wanting to do a heart transplant as a kind of national status symbol. I have very little doubt that this is worth carrying on with when we know more about tissue immunology and the means of resisting the rejection of tissues, and it may well be that in ten years' time, this operation will not merit even a word in a newspaper; it will be done routinely. I think surrounding circumstances have led many people to have second thoughts about its advisability. Also one must realise that it may well be that there will be no transplants in the sense of organ transplants, but various types of mechanical devices will enable us to carry on.

With regard to euthanasia, I should just like to tell you one story. There was a very distinguished professor who made his doctor promise him that if he ever suffered from an incurable disease he would give him an injection to end his life. Well alas, this distinguished professor did develop a very grave disease. And he then refused to have any injections whatsoever from the doctor lest it was the final one. This is one reason why I see very grave objections to the legalisation of euthanasia. I think that all doctors would agree that their duty is to relieve pain and, if in the course of that, a dose of the pain-relieving drug which they are administering happened to prove fatal to the patient, well, that would be unfortunate. But deliberately to do so and for it to be known that the law permits it, would, it seems to me, undermine that trust which should exist between doctor and patient. And most of my colleagues, I know, would be strongly opposed to the legalisation of voluntary euthanasia.

II ABORTION

T. N. A. JEFFCOATE & PHILIPPA FOOT

JEFFCOATE Abortion means the termination of pregnancy either naturally, which is common, or unnaturally, which is less common, before the foetus or child is viable; that is, capable of living independently of its mother. Any child of less than 28 weeks' maturity is arbitrarily defined by legal statute as being non-viable. Unfortunately, some babies are ignorant of the law and, having been born after only 25, 26 or 27 weeks' development, proceed to survive. They are then registered as members of the community which denies that they can exist. Babies born much earlier, say after twelve weeks' development, have all their organs fully formed, and show signs – such as physical movement, nerve reflexes and heartbeat – which in the adult would be accepted as certain evidence of life. Even at six weeks the heart of a foetus is beating regularly and strongly. An immediate problem, therefore, is to decide whether induction of abortion means the destruction of a living person – and this in turn involves defining life. This seems to me even more difficult than defining death, a matter which, with the development of transplant operations, becomes increasingly controversial. The ovum, even before fertilisation, is a living structure, but few would regard it as a human being. But what of the fully-formed and active foetus of 12 weeks' development, or the one aged 26 weeks which, despite the law, is sometimes viable? In the previous section the main contributors expressed the view that a viable baby still alive in the uterus after its mother's death deserves as much care from the doctor to ensure its survival as if it were already born. This appears to confer on the baby *in utero* the rights of citizenship.

The definition of human life is a matter for philosophers and I leave it to Mrs Foot. Nevertheless it should be noted that, in these days when childbearing is so safe for the mother, the modern obstetrician devotes an increasing amount of time and skill to caring for the unborn foetus which to him is a patient whose welfare is his prime concern. The normal woman, too, regards the young embryo inside her uterus as a very real person. If she suffers spontaneous, let alone induced, abortion her sensation of loss is almost as real as if one of her children is taken from her. This is true even though, prior to its conception and prior to its expulsion, the pregnancy was unwanted.

The Abortion Act 1967 was designed from the outset to be unsatisfactory in that the original Bill was sponsored by a small but strongly organised band of agitators who, whilst having to disguise their real objective, swayed public and parliamentary opinion by propaganda and misrepresentation of the position existing at the time; they aroused emotions by fantasy rather than fact. For example, they multiplied the number of criminal abortions in this country by at least ten, to produce the absurd figure of 250,000 a year. They talked of large numbers of young healthy women dying at the hands of criminal abortionists, when the *known* figure for fatal cases – mostly amongst middle-aged married women who operated on themselves – was only between twenty and thirty each year. The final effect of this sort of distortion of fact and purpose, and of inevitable compromise, was an Act, the wording of which is, in part at least, beyond rational interpretation. Thus, one clause permits the termination of pregancy if two registered medical practitioners are of the opinion that 'the continuance of pregnancy would involve risk to the life of the pregnant woman or of injury to the physical or mental health of the pregnant woman, *or any existing children of her family*, greater than if the pregnancy were terminated.' Regulations governing the Act define 'children of the family' as meaning natural, adopted, fostered or step-children, up to the age of sixteen years. This means that doctors are now being asked to decide whether the physical and mental benefits of performing an operation on one person are less than the nebulous ones to which a third person, such as a step-son aged fifteen years, might be exposed by having a half-brother.

In the hope of avoiding such anomalies, and of making the Abortion Act workable and valuable to the community, all the professional medical bodies in this country repeatedly offered help at the time it was being formulated, and they spoke with one voice. Such advice was, in the main, disregarded. Indeed, it was reported that during the Committee Stage of the Bill one Member of Parliament said, 'We are not here to listen to professional advice and opinion. We are here to legislate.' This attitude is another example of what is now widely recognised as a political threat to all professions. It is part of a trend which aims to weaken the position of independent informed opinion. In regard to abortion the attack still continues. Those who failed by way of the wording of the Act to make it impossible for a doctor to be directed to operate against his better judgement are now occupied in moulding public opinion on the interpretation of its clauses. Newspaper columnists outline the circumstances under which any woman can *demand* an abortion, choosing and repeating words such as 'demand' so that the public is misled. Paid for by money coming from overseas, a pamphlet was produced in this country and widely circulated, a pamphlet that aims by selective emphasis to guide doctors about the new indications for abortion.

The truth is that, except for its confused reference to other children of the family, the Abortion Act of 1967 leaves the indications for terminating pregnancy unchanged. The old law, which makes it a criminal offence to induce or to attempt to induce abortion illegally, is still in force. The new law merely states the circumstances under which it is legally *permissible* to terminate a pregnancy. It is permissive and not mandatory. It allows the doctor what he had previously, namely a wide range of freedom in reaching his personal opinion of what is best from the standpoint of protecting the physical and mental health of his woman patient. It also lists what was hitherto an implied and accepted indication for abortion, namely the real likelihood of the child being born with disabilities so great as not to permit it to enjoy its subsequent existence. There is no provision for terminating pregnancy on social grounds alone, although environmental factors are necessarily taken into consideration, and always have been, by any doctor when judging the effect of pregnancy on health. Psychiatric indications remain as previously; some genuine, some existing only in the imagination.

The Abortion Act now clearly lays down the need for a doctor, when recommending or performing abortion, to be satisfied that this surgical procedure is safer than the continuance of pregnancy in that particular case. Those who repeatedly state that induction of abortion under modern conditions is without hazard, generally quote figures which come from behind the Iron Curtain and which are politically adjusted. Do any of us believe accounts of the invasion of Czechoslovakia put out by Russia and her satellites? The official reports of their experience with legalised abortion are equally unreliable. Thus the Government returns of one country indicate that, during 1966, 90,000 abortions were induced with the patient under general anaesthesia and this without a single death. Every anaesthetist knows that, even without counting risks of the operation itself, it is impossible to administer such a large number of general anaesthetics without fatal mishaps. If one talks to gynaecologists from Hungary and Czechoslovakia, when they are in this country and free to tell the truth, they present a different story, one which fits with all other professional experience. They admit that deaths occur, that the uterus is ruptured once in every 250 cases, that significant illness follows in three to fifteen per cent of cases, that one or two per cent of women are subsequently sterile, and that young girls often have their future reproductive careers prejudiced by immunisation to rhesus factor and by injuries to the uterus which mean that all their subsequent pregnancies end in abortion or stillbirth. The truth is, as far as one can obtain it, that abortion carried out on healthy women probably carries a mortality rate of at least 0·3 per 1,000, which is as high as the maternal mortality rate (including criminal abortions) in this country.

The healthy unmarried girl with an unwanted pregnancy may present a picture which arouses sympathy and a desire to protect her from the embarrassment of having a child. Yet a gynaecologist who has her real interests at heart may hesitate to induce abortion when he knows that the ultimate effect may be to ruin her later life by childlessness if not major ill-health. The psychological consequences of abortion to the woman are more difficult to assess, but it is accepted that a significant proportion of women – sometimes rated as twenty to thirty per cent in the past – are adversely affected emotionally throughout their life.

One can understand some women, with their new emancipation, taking the view that they themselves should decide whether their pregnancy should be terminated or not; that they should have the right to demand its removal. If there were an acceptable method of inducing abortion which they themselves could employ I can see no reason why they should not be free to do so, providing they appreciated the risks. There may come a time when an efficient oral abortifacient is discovered. A woman might then choose to take this, just as she can now elect to take oral contraceptives or to smoke cigarettes, despite any hazards involved. Meanwhile, however, abortion necessitates an operation, carried out by a skilled team, consisting of surgeon, anaesthetist, and nurses. These are all motivated by a strong ethical code and are dedicated to protect life and health. Only they can form a detached and professional opinion as to what is in the best interests of the patient.

Now what has been the effect of the Abortion Act 1967 and of all the discussion which it has aroused? It was reported in the House of Commons in early October 1968, that during five months since the Act came into force, 13,000 abortions had been notified. Moreover, as we expected, these have involved a certain number of deaths. If the practice is continued at this level it means a total of 30,000 induced abortions a year in England and Wales.[1] The returns also show that forty per cent of these abortions, that is 10,000 per annum, are being performed in the relatively small number of private nursing homes licensed for the purpose, in which only a relatively small number of doctors operate, and then for fees. So it would seem that the Act has already had the effect, which was predicted, of legalising and encouraging the very activities which its sponsors claimed it would suppress.

Has criminal abortion been eliminated by the Act? This was another declared object of those who wanted the law reformed. No one yet knows what has happened in this respect, but every other country which has legalised abortion has found that the result, initially at least, is not to decrease the number of criminal abortions; often it has increased it. Abortion, like crime and sex, is encouraged when it is advertised by way of mass media publicity. The community comes to regard it as acceptable, if not proper. Even courts of law change their attitude and so lighten the penalties that the criminal abortionist is no longer deterred. Changes in public conscience, for good or evil according to the outlook of each one of us individually, are already becoming evident. The number of abortions induced in National Health Service hospitals is now six times more than it was in 1964, and three times more than in 1966. So some, if not all, doctors have been adopting an increasingly liberal attitude during

[1] Statistics covering the first year of the working of the Act confirm this figure.

the last five years. This again may be quite proper and in keeping with changing times. It is for each doctor to judge what is best in each case, and there is room for wide differences of opinion. Yet there is no doubt that many of the younger members of the medical profession, those whose economic and professional positions are not secure, are being coerced into terminating pregnancy when they themselves can find little justification for so doing. Some shrug their shoulders and find it easier, even if distasteful, to bow to public and political pressures than to apply their professional knowledge. Some are fearful that if they follow their conscience, they may put their future careers in peril; others that the new Act exposes them to possible legal action if they refuse a request for abortion. Are we approaching a situation, which already obtains in many European countries, where the doctor employed by the State has to perform operations which he regards as unethical, otherwise he loses his employment?

Whether doctors are now taking a more liberal view of abortion because their honest opinion is changing, or because of outside pressures, the fact remains that more and more women are being admitted to our hospitals for the purpose of having a pregnancy terminated. If this is to be done with maximum safety, it has to be arranged at the earliest possible moment, so feckless girls and women with unwanted pregnancies have to be admitted as a matter of urgency, taking precedence over women anxiously waiting to have their prolapse, or other disability, cured. Is it right that the promiscuous girl, who has not troubled to practise contraception, should have priority over the decent married woman, who has been waiting perhaps twelve months for admission for investigation of sterility?

I offer one final line of thought. Approximately eight per cent of married couples in this country prove to be permanently sterile, despite treatment. Many of these now satisfy their parental instincts and enjoy life to its full by adopting one or more children. Such children are mostly the result of unwanted pregnancies, and already there are insufficient to satisfy demand. How great is the threat to the happiness of countless members of our community if all unwanted pregnancies are removed at the outset? Again, is it in the interests of a ten-week-old foetus to be destroyed, because someone considers that its natural mother may not give it good attention after birth? Or is it better for it to be born in the expectation, or even certainty, that it will receive loving and devoted care from a couple who will never have a child of their own?

FOOT Professor Jeffcoate has discussed some medical and legal aspects of abortion. I must talk about the morality of it, and I should say right from the beginning that I regard this as a dreadfully difficult thing to have to do. The topic of abortion is extraordinarily complex and perplexing from a moral philosopher's point of view, and it is very hard to see one's way around it clearly enough to talk any sense.

Let me start by saying what is obvious enough: that there is a strong moral case for the termination of a pregnancy in some sad cases; for what hangs on it may be, for instance, the saving of the mother's life, or her health, or the avoidance of great unhappiness, and in general we have a positive duty to do the things that are necessary for such good ends. It is only because it is not clear whether we have the right to do this thing, to destroy the foetus, even for such an end, that a doubt can arise at all. That we do elsewhere recognise the limitations of the means that may be taken even to a good end is certain, since we do not, for instance, think it right to kill anyone in the interests of cancer research, even if the lives of a lot of people could be saved. And what we must decide is whether abortion is, or is not, another case like this. Everything hangs on the difference, or lack of difference, between terminating a pregnancy and killing a human being, so I would put the dilemma as follows: Either the foetus is to be seen as a human being, or it is not. If it is a human being, then in destroying it one kills a human being, in which case very few abortions can be said to be justified, and not many of those which were permitted under the old legislation, even before the Bourne case had made it unnecessary to show that the mother's life was actually in danger. For while we would be horrified at the idea that we could kill a small child to spare his mother ill-health we do not think it morally permissible to kill one person even to save the life of another. So on the thesis that the foetus has the full status of a human being there would, I think, be only one allowable case of abortion: where the mother was in danger and the child could not in any case be born alive. There are, of course, some Catholics who dispute the morality of the directly intended destruction of the foetus even in such circumstances, which seems to me quite unreasonable. But to allow abortion in such cases where the child could not survive, would be only a slight mitigation of the extreme position that we are now considering.

Let me return to the dilemma. Either, I said, the foetus is counted as a human being, in which case the extreme consequences follow, and hardly any abortion can be justified, or else it is not. If it is not, then either of two things may again be said. Either we may think of ourselves as having some duties towards the foetus as a potential human being, so that we do not have the right to destroy it except in grave circumstances, or we may think that we have the right to perform an abortion whenever we choose. Even on the third and last view the moral issue is not closed, and it does not follow that everyone would choose abortion rather than suffer hardship. For even if one thinks that one has the *right* to do this, one might reject the idea of abortion, because it is natural to think of the unborn child as something marvellous and precious and not to be exchanged for such a thing as a respectable position in society or an uninterrupted career. There can be an assertion of moral values in the decision about abortion, even if rights and duties are not thought to exist, and it is perhaps useful to say this to explain why even those who do not think of abortion as infringing the rights of the unborn may nevertheless feel that the refusal of an abortion can be something rather important from the moral point of view. For us, however, the crucial question is whether one actually has the right to demand, or perform, an abortion and to this difficult question I must return.

Is a human foetus a human being or not? Arguing on one side, we can point out that it is natural to talk of a particular human being in the early stage of its development when what we mean is the foetus, and here we will be carrying the notion of this human being back behind the moment of birth. On the other hand, we might say that the foetus is no more a human being at the time it is a foetus than an acorn is an oak tree when it is still an acorn. What is interesting is that it is a bit more natural to carry the idea of a human being back to the foetus stage and even to that of the very early embryo, than it is to think of an acorn being an oak tree. So it would not perhaps seem totally whimsical to count a pregnant mother for two if counting the human beings in a room, though there wouldn't seem anything to force us into doing so. And here, it seems to me, is the odd truth of the matter. For it looks as if we do have alternative criteria of what we shall count as a human being, and that at least two of these are both allowable. So we might say that any individual thing that will develop into a being with human characteristics is a human being, and that we have no right to do to it what we have no right to do to a human being; or we might say that nothing can be a human being until it has a specifically human kind of existence, i.e. a life that is separate.

Separate existence does, of course, carry a lot with it, since the unborn child cannot be looked after, as even the smallest baby may be, with an affectionate response to the signs of its needs. I mean to say that it is not a superficial matter, separate existence, which we find it convenient to stress. Both of these criteria of the human being, the potentiality and the separate existence seem to me allowable. What would, on the other hand, be strange would be to insist that a human being was what looked like a human being, since size and shape are not very important parts of our concept of a human being. Human beings might come in different shapes and sizes, far more than they do, so long as a human form of life was maintained. It would seem odd, therefore, to make a distinction between early and late abortion on the ground that after a time the foetus has the shape of a human being, and I don't myself see how one could make such a distinction at all, unless perhaps one separated off the viable foetus because it can have an independent life. If Professor Jeffcoate asks me to say when we first exist as a human being, or a person, I should say either from the moment of conception, because of the potentiality of this individual thing for developing into a human child, or else from the time of viability or birth, because it is then that a separate human life begins. The uncomfortable part of this conclusion is that there seem to be no criteria for deciding which way we shall apply our concept of a human being. Neither seems to do violence to our concepts in the way in which, for instance, violence is done to the concept of *killing* if one tries to apply it to the prevention of conception, or again to the concept of a *human being* if one says that people of some different race are not human. I am inclined to think that one must recognise a genuine subjectivity about the decision as to whether to count a foetus as a human being and accord it human rights, and that in this respect the issue of abortion is unlike many other moral issues. I myself would say it is legitimate to see the foetus as not a human being and not having rights, and, therefore, that abortion should be permitted because of the misery that is otherwise going to exist. That there is such misery is partly a function of our rotten society, with its censoriousness towards the unmarried mother, and its isolated, defensive, ungenerous way of living. But some abortions would be needed to avoid human unhappiness even in a better society than ours.

Those are the remarks that I wanted to make on the general topic, but I should like to say one or two things, off the cuff, in reply to Professor Jeffcoate, and you must forgive me if these are a little stumbling. First of all I doubt if the question about the definition of life is very important, since it is clear that in the very early stage we are dealing with a living organism, but one that is not necessarily to be counted a human being. Then, secondly, Professor Jeffcoate did seem to me to underestimate the evils that the new Act was designed to mitigate. He spoke about the dangers of even the best abortion, and thought that the number of deaths from back-street abortions had been overestimated. But after all death was not the only evil involved. The misery suffered by girls in the hands of back-street abortionists and the kind of people who would send them to back-street abortionists, was very great indeed, even if there was no physical damage, and of course there often was. I don't think anybody who has seen anything of this could dispute what I say. Thirdly, I agree that the new Act has farcical results, for I believe it is always possible to find a doctor who will certify that the continuance of the pregnancy will involve risks to the mental health of the pregnant woman or her family, and it seems rather a farce that this form should be gone through and that we should be pretending to give some protection to the unborn while not actually doing it. Then, fourthly, I am a little puzzled about Professor Jeffcoate's own position. I cannot quite make out what his objections to abortion are. He says that if abortion were (a) safe and (b) self-administered there would be no objection to it, but I did not quite understand about the self-administration. Is this because he doesn't want the time of doctors to be taken in this business when they should be doing other things? If this is it, one would point out, as it has often been pointed out before, that the birth of a child needs more hospital time, and can as little wait, as the termination of the pregnancy; but perhaps that was not his point, and he has some other reason for requiring self-administration. I don't myself see why, if there is no objection to the woman terminating her own pregnancy, there should be an objection to the doctor doing so; because surely if there is an objection to the doctor doing so it should be because it is a case of taking life, and if it is a case of taking life there should be an objection to the woman doing so as well. And, finally, perhaps Professor Jeffcoate would forgive me if I take exception to his remark about the promiscuous girl when he is talking about an unmarried mother. I don't know why he should assume that every girl who gets pregnant without being married is promiscuous.

JEFFCOATE In many of the medical and moral aspects of the issues which face society today, the doctor and the philosopher seem to me to go hand in hand. This applies, for example, to sexual permissiveness. Incidentally, Mrs Foot, I wasn't suggesting that all unmarried mothers are promiscuous. I merely took a particular instance. A few of them, at least, are promiscuous; as the following episode which happened recently in a Liverpool hospital shows. A girl, aged fifteen, reported pregnant and met a rather sympathetic gynaecologist who terminated the pregnancy. She was back in six months quite unconcernedly asking for a second abortion. So the gynaecologist chatted to this girl and said, 'Well now look, you really can't carry on like this, you're running great risks. You're running risks of getting venereal disease. You really must change your ways of living.' So the girl said, 'Very well,' got up from the couch and, as she was leaving the room, turned with a smile to the gynaecologist and asked, 'Can you give up smoking?'

What I had in mind was that there are certain matters, like sexual freedom, which both the philosopher and the doctor may well come to regard as acceptable. They perhaps can both accept it as part of the evolution of society. The doctor may not only accept this as being morally right, he can very well take every opportunity to provide contraceptive advice for all and sundry, including the unmarried, and this may be quite correct. Indeed, and certainly as far as the gynaecologists are concerned, our emphasis has always been on prevention rather than cure. It always seems to us better to provide means of contraception which is a relatively harmless proceeding for anyone who wishes it, than to engage in the wholesale termination of pregnancies which is not a harmless procedure. Abortion is a threat to life and health. And there is an ethical difficulty when it comes to terminating an unwanted pregnancy. Even if an abortion is morally acceptable, even if we can prove that we're not destroying another individual, the carrying out of abortion at present involves a third person – third in addition to the mother and the child. I suggested that I could well see a case, if there were an efficient method, for women deciding themselves to take an abortifacient because this would not involve a third person. Nurses as well as doctors, already dedicated to saving life and health and having a strong ethical code, find it objectionable to terminate a pregnancy unless they are completely convinced that it is in the interests of the physical, or mental, health of the woman. Some people may say, 'Oh well, medical ethics are old-fashioned and out-of-date and we shouldn't be bothered with them in these days.' So perhaps I might just emphasise that the whole concept of medical ethics is not basically in the interests of the medical profession; it is in the interests of the patient and the community. In other words it sets a standard of conduct, which the doctor must follow, which is vital to ensuring the continuance of the doctor/patient relationship; without this strong code of professional ethics, patients would lose faith in their doctors.

FOOT I am a little puzzled about what Professor Jeffcoate means. I am not clear whether the difficulty is that there is a third person, or that he is a doctor. I don't see why a third person should make any difference if the action is not bad.

JEFFCOATE As things stand at present the third person concerned in inducing an abortion must be a doctor, a trained surgeon, and his training and outlook makes abortion unethical unless there is a good medical indication of its necessity. If society wants abortion on demand, then it should perhaps look to some other form of third person. After all we used to have a public executioner. Couldn't we have public abortionists? Couldn't we have abortionaria instead of hospitals in which the work would be done? In fact these exist in certain countries in the world.

COHEN I think we ought to remind ourselves what are the provisions of the Abortion Act, and I took it on myself to write them down, as I suspected that there might be some deviation from the actual phrases used in the Abortion Act, and Professor Jeffcoate has once or twice, I suspect, dealt with something which is not in the Abortion Act.

The Abortion Act states that it is legal to perform an abortion if two registered medical practitioners in good faith are of opinion firstly, that the continuance of pregnancy would involve risk to the life of the pregnant woman, or injury to her physical or mental health, or to any existing child, greater than if pregnancy were terminated and secondly, if there is a substantial risk that, if the child were born, it would suffer from such physical or mental defect as to be seriously handicapped. I think it's only right to say that when Professor Jeffcoate states that the Abortion Act of 1967 leaves the indications of terminating pregnancy exactly as they were before, that just is not accurate, because certainly before the Rex *v.* Bourne Case, in 1937, no one in this country knew what the law permitted in regard to abortion. And in that case the judge said that if there were danger to the life of the mother (he said to the health, but after all health implies life), then an abortion may be carried out without its being a criminal offence. But I do not know of any case before 1937 in which any similar decision was taken.

The Abortion Act – and I am not at the moment supporting it or saying that it is something which ought not to have been passed – is perfectly clear that doctors must act in good faith; that is to say, that they in good faith believe (which may be difficult to prove, or disprove) that there is a danger to the physical or mental health of the mother, or that there is a risk that a child will be born deformed to such a degree that he will survive with a grave disability. That is the situation, and I think we must bear that in mind in discussing the legal position.

This does not involve the moral dilemma. This is a permissive Act. No doctor need undertake an abortion if he has a conscientious objection to so doing. No patient need have an abortion if she has any conscientious objection, or wishes to continue to have a live child. But the provisions of the Act are clear – although it is true, as has been said, that in some instances it may prove a little difficult to interpret them.

JEFFCOATE You are right to point out that prior to 1938, prior to the Rex *v.* Bourne Case, the situation was very different. But as a result of that case, and as a result of several other cases, the case law was such that, in practice, the indications for terminating pregnancy, not in 1937, but in 1967, before the present Act came into force, were exactly the same as they are now. In other words, there was no act which said: 'You can terminate a pregnancy if the baby is at serious risk of being malformed', but every gynaecologist, or other doctor concerned, recognised that if there was a real hazard of the baby being affected the mother was then so worried that she was psychologically disturbed; we then had a wonderful psychiatric indication for terminating the pregnancy. So, in fact, the practice of last year was exactly the same as this year. We had nothing in writing to guide us but we had case law on which to depend.

COHEN But you might well have been called upon to defend such an action.

JEFFCOATE Oh yes, and this is the one great difference made by the new law. Prior to the Abortion Act the doctor or gynaecologist was free to interpret the situation very widely – but his conduct was always controlled by the knowledge that if anyone doubted the propriety of his termination of a pregnancy, he might have to defend his action in that particular case. What the new law has done is to remove that safeguard.

The Chairman then opened the discussion to the audience and invited them to put questions to the speakers.

D. CALDWELL Would Professor Jeffcoate not agree that one new factor in the Act is the registration of abortion, which was not compulsory before? And does he envisage the registration being analysed by some panel of gynaecologists in pay of the Ministry of Health who, if they do find cases in which women die following abortion carried out on flimsy grounds, will advise reform so that there will be better legislation promulgated in the future?

JEFFCOATE I think the second question could probably only be answered by the Chief Medical Officer of the Ministry. But you have raised a point of some interest, and importance, namely, that under the new Act not only do certificates have to be signed before abortion is induced, but abortion becomes a notifiable condition. Some people have taken an adverse view of this, but it seems to me that this is a very wise provision. Before this Act, no one really knew how many abortions occurred in this country; we knew how many babies were born because they were all registered, but we did not know how many women aborted. We certainly did not know exactly how many criminal abortions were carried out and any assessment was made indirectly on evidence collected from various souces. So I think it is very important that, if we are going to liberalise abortion, there should be accurate records kept as to what is going on – how many operations are being done, and what are their hazards. At the moment I say that termination of pregnancy is a potentially dangerous operation; somebody else says it is completely free from risk. It would be right to have statistics, and this is the purpose of notification.

D. B. BARNETT I would like to ask Professor Jeffcoate about the psychological trauma and guilt complexes which women have once their pregnancies have been terminated, and how can one assess this factor?

JEFFCOATE This again is difficult. Studies have been made, mostly in Scandinavia, of women who have had abortions induced on what are euphemistically called humane grounds. Some of these reports go back many years, and may be out-of-date. But the sort of figures that are given are something like twenty-five to thirty per cent of women being adversely affected in the sense that they have permanent regrets that the abortion was induced. A smaller percentage are seriously affected. But the criteria for judgement of the results must be very fluid and are often matters of opinion. This is one of the great difficulties of the present situation in this country. There are many doctors who are recommending abortion, even to the extent of signing certificates; a psychiatrist might do it, or a physician, or a surgeon. But the majority of these doctors never see the patients again, and they have no idea what happens psychologically, either when their advice is accepted or when it is over-ruled. They really do not know what happens if abortion is induced or if the pregnancy is allowed to go on. The ultimate effect is that quoted results may represent little more than guesswork and opinion.

P. HARPER I am a psychiatrist. Professor Jeffcoate cites, as a wonderful example of a valid psychiatric indication for termination of a pregnancy, a mother's fear of a deformed baby from rubella; and in the main context of his paper he mentioned psychiatric indications, some of which are real and some of which exist only in the imagination. I wonder could he give us an example of the latter, and how did he distinguish?

JEFFCOATE Well, I said this because at the present time any woman with an unwanted pregnancy has, unless she is physically ill, to produce a psychiatric reason for terminating pregnancy, if the operation is to be lawful. And this may mean stretching the psychiatric reasons. Take, for example, an unmarried girl who finds herself pregnant and doesn't want to be. Or the woman of forty who thinks her family is complete and then to her horror finds herself pregnant again. In both these cases the patient is naturally very upset. Now the fact that they are distressed to find themselves in this embarrassing situation is the very proof that their psyche is completely normal. This is a normal reaction; it proves that the woman's psyche is normal, yet many argue that it is a psychiatric indication for terminating pregnancy.

L. RATOFF I am a general practitioner. Could I just follow this one point by asking whether anybody has considered that the unwanted pregnancies may well be deep psychological disorders in themselves, and that the abortion is the removing of a symptom without in fact curing the underlying psychological disease.

JEFFCOATE I think there is something in this. There is a certain class of woman who deliberately likes to take the risk of becoming pregnant. She will deliberately avoid practising contraception, even if unmarried. This in itself may be evidence of some psychological upset, but I would not know the details of it. It is the psychiatrist's field.

FOOT Might I just make an obvious remark. Surely one would want to remove the symptom as well. I mean, there is no argument for not curing the symptom just because you are not curing the disease.

SHEILA DONNELLAN I am a social worker and very often have to deal with girls who are pregnant and advise them about what they can do if they continue with their pregnancy. Now does Professor Jeffcoate ever see the girls who have to go on with pregnancy and who suffer tremendous heartbreak, and very often psychological trauma, as a result of having to part with their babies for adoption? Also I would question most sincerely his comment about keeping the supply of unwanted babies to satisfy the demands of childless couples. A large number of the young people whom I have to see are adopted children who themselves have never come to terms with being adopted.

JEFFCOATE It may well be that adoption is not the answer to all the problems of the unwanted child, either for the child or for natural and adopting parents. I merely put forward a line of thought; do we really want to have no unwanted babies in the country? I agree that unmarried girls who go on with their pregnancy may suffer as much psychological upset as if they had had the pregnancy terminated. And there are some who are heartbroken by having to give up their baby to be adopted. They are probably the very ones who would have been heartbroken if the pregnancy had been terminated. Maternal instinct can be so strong that the loss of a baby by either abortion or adoption is equally distressing.

C. TAYLOR I have been heartened by the comments of Mrs Foot that this is very much an area for subjective opinion and this encourages me in the attitudes I have taken because I think general practitioners are more exposed to subjectivity in this field than perhaps any other section of the profession. Whilst appreciating the problems of consultant colleagues, I hope they appreciate even more the problems of their general practitioner colleagues. I would ask whether our speakers agree that we are suffering at present from exacerbation of the situation, which may before long settle down to some sort of normality, particularly with the spread of birth control advice. I commend Professor Jeffcoate for his courageous statement that birth control advice should be freely available to all who seek it, irrespective of their status. Regrettably this is not particularly easy for the unmarried in this city of Liverpool. I recall a case which was a challenge to my profession. A girl, with a serious and very stable relationship and not promiscuous but not contemplating marriage, went to her general practitioner for birth control advice and was refused this. She then went to a hospital outpatient department, regrettably on the wrong day, and was refused advice. Then, with tremendous courage, I think, for a nervous single young student, went to a Clinic – again unfortunately just a few weeks before their policy to the unmarried changed. So she did not get the advice, and she became pregnant. I don't think a person can demonstrate much more strongly that they are anxious to avoid a pregnancy. I know bad cases make bad law, but does Professor Jeffcoate think that, in all cases where pregnancy arises as a result of the failure of our colleagues to give the necessary advice, we as a profession have any additional responsibility in the matter of considering termination?

JEFFCOATE I would find it very difficult to take on responsibilities which really belong to someone else. I think your comment that some of our present problems may represent a temporary emotional upsurge, and that this may all settle, could well be true, because there is no doubt that a lot of the discussions that have gone on, and a lot of the statements that have been made, have all been motivated and twisted. So they have aroused very natural emotional reactions in all of us and this makes it difficult to be scientific. I think every individual has an emotional approach to this subject deep down. They try and keep it deep down, and let science come on top, but this is not easy.

FOOT I couldn't agree more with what the questioner said and with Professor Jeffcoate's stand about contraception. It does seem to me that this is not a subjective matter. There is a plain duty to provide contraceptive advice and to avoid the present demand for abortion with the misery that is entailed. I think that people do go to town on the wrong things, morally speaking, and that this is exactly the kind of thing on which they should take a strong moral stand.

J. PINSENT I would like to ask if our speakers would discuss the whole moral question of medical ethics? It seems to me that much of the discussion is about who is entitled to decide what. Some people would say that if I wish some professional to do something for me I have the right to go to him and say: 'Do it for me.' Another view might be that the individual doctor must decide: I may refuse his advice but I cannot ask him to do something for me. I would be interested to hear what both speakers think about the moral criteria by which questions like this should be decided. My instinct is to feel that there are many matters that I should decide for myself.

COHEN But surely what you decide for yourself is to seek a doctor's advice. If you do this then you can either reject or accept the advice he gives you. But you cannot demand that he should do something which he is unwilling to do, any more than you can demand it of any other person. In the case of the doctor, he expresses his professional view and gives you advice which it is for you to accept or reject. But you cannot say to him, 'You must operate on my appendix,' or 'You must amputate my left leg' if he says that neither your appendix nor your left leg are in any way diseased or require amputation.

Perhaps I ought to have a final word or two. I think it is abundantly clear from what Professor Jeffcoate has said that his objections to the Abortion Act are essentially medical – the surgical risks of abortion. If there were a safe pill, *pilula uteri evacuans* I suppose, we can see no reason why abortion should not be allowed, provided that the risks are appreciated. He argues that abortion is continuing to increase but he said later that this may possibly be a temporary phase. However, he made his case clear that on medical grounds he thought that there were certain aspects of the Abortion Act which were unsatisfactory, that the wording was somewhat loose and that it might have to be tightened up. Mrs Foot deals with the issue from the moral or philosophical standpoint. She quite rightly said that the definition of life is not terribly relevant to the problem which confronts us. After all, a virus is living, the single cell is living, a multi-cellular organism is living, an organism higher up the evolutionary scale is living. All these are manifestations of the noun 'life'. And the question then becomes, certainly a foetus is living in the sense that it has life, but has it the full status of a human being? She approached this with a philosophical clarity, which I am sure we all appreciated. And she came to the conclusion that it is perhaps legitimate to perform abortion in the medium of our rotten society, but some abortions would be justified even in a better society. This was a subjective decision which we should each take on whatever may be the grounds that decide us.

III CONTRACEPTION

H. H. FRANCIS & G. R. DUNSTAN

FRANCIS I believe that coitus without efficient contraception is irresponsible and anti-social in all pre-marital and extra-marital affairs and after the birth of the third child within marriage. I would define the pill, coil, diaphragm, and sheath as efficient methods of contraception with the addition of tubal ligation and vasotomy for couples with three living children.

We are in the midst of a unique demographic crisis, an explosion of the world population. With 110 million births each year, humans are increasing by 60 million every year, that is, by more than the entire population of the United Kingdom. The world population has doubled since the 1914–18 War, and if present trends continue it will double again before the end of this century. In contrast, the surface area of the earth is finite and static, 52 million square miles with only one-third potentially usable. It is already supporting a total population of 3,500 million at a density of 60 people per square mile overall, or 180 per usable square mile. The size of any population is determined by three factors: birth rate, death rate, and migration. Under primitive conditions man has a birth rate of 40 per thousand total population per year, balanced by a death rate of 40 per thousand per year. The birth rate in developing countries still approximates to 40 but the death rate, as a result of advances in preventive and therapeutic medicine, is 20 per thousand. This gives a crude rate of increase of 20 per thousand, or 2 per cent per year. As an example of how public health successes bring their own problems, Ceylon launched a nation-wide attack on the mosquito in 1946. Within one decade the human death rate was cut in half, but the birth rate remained unchanged and the population of Ceylon increased by 80 per cent. The developed nations have lowered their birth rates to 20 per thousand per year, but the wider and more intensive application of preventive medicine and advances in therapy have reduced their death rates to 10 per thousand, giving an annual growth of 10 per thousand, or 1 per cent. The present global figures are, birth 34 per thousand, death 16 per thousand, giving an increase of 18 per thousand per annum or 1·8 per cent. This will lead to doubling of the world population every 30 years. Demographic trends become comprehensible when likened to motoring: a rate of increase is equivalent to acceleration and the size of a population to the distance travelled.

It should not be concluded that the developing countries alone are in need of population control. Current rates of increase must be considered against the background of existing densities of population. England and Wales is the third most densely populated area in the world, if we exclude small enclaves and islands with obvious geographic limitations, such as Hong Kong, Singapore, Mauritius and Gibraltar. Holland leads the world with 960 persons per square mile. Taiwan, better known as Formosa, is second with 925, while England and Wales are third with 830 persons per square mile. The total populations of these three countries are: 11, 13 and 49 millions respectively, so if density and total population are compounded, England and Wales is 'top of the pops'. In addition, the population of England and Wales is increasing by one-third of a million annually, a rate of increase of 0·8 per cent. This is as serious as the increment of 2·4 per cent each year in India which has only 420 persons per square mile, or 2·1 per cent increase in Pakistan with 280 people per square mile. It is all the less excusable in that the citizens of this country have adequate social security, whereas members of emergent countries must beget several sons to ensure that their own family unit can provide food and shelter in sickness and old age. Furthermore, in 1955, when most Western countries were reducing their birth rates, England and Wales embarked upon an orgy of reproduction. Live births rose from 670,000 to 870,000 by 1964. At that time doctors who were demographically aware took alarm, realising that children born during the much publicised 'first bulge' were approaching the peak reproductive age of 20 to 25 years. With pill, coil, and ligature, annual births were reduced to 810,000 by 1967 but this was still 150,000 above the average for this century. The 'second bulge' is due in part to reduction in the age of bride and groom by one and a quarter years per decade since the second war, as the ultimate size of family is inversely proportional to age at marriage. This trend is, of course, not unique to this country because in the United States 40 per cent of brides are teenaged.

Another disturbing feature in Britain is the increase in illegitimate births. Whereas 31,000 illegitimate births occurred in England and Wales in 1955, there were 67,000 in 1967; 8 per cent of all live births. The adoption market, a sensitive barometer of the national economy, cannot absorb an illegitimate birth rate of more than 10 per cent even in times of plenty. Whereas the legitimate birth rate has fallen since 1964, no such trend is apparent among births to the unmarried in this country. We may see surplus children spending their childhood in orphanages as in New Zealand, which has the highest illegitimate birth rate among developed countries, namely 13 per cent. In England and Wales 67,000 illegitimate births represent 20 per cent of the 330,000 births which must be eliminated each year if we are to stabilise the population.

Lest any should believe that 'everyone is welcome on Earth and the more the merrier', let us consider the spacial, medical, and economic ill-effects of over-population. The supply of fresh water becomes critical long before food shortages arise. Many of the world's large cities, such as New York, have a persistent shortage of water but rarely of food. New York's grubby buses already bear the sign 'We are not washing so that you can'. The difficulty of keeping sewage and drinking water apart has brought typhoid back to Europe in the 1960s. This is the age of effluence, with man, the dirtiest animal on Earth, progressively making a slum of nature. Rivers everywhere are polluted in greater or less degree and the sea has become the waste-pipe of the world. One cannot even swim off the coast of England, although one can go through the motions of it. London draws two-thirds of its water supply from a river which contains the purified sewage of Swindon, Oxford, and Reading. The Welsh Nationalists who repeatedly blow up the mains bringing water to Liverpool would be better advised to preach family planning at the Pier Head. Those who oppose the enclosure of yet another lake in Westmorland as a water reservoir should attack the problem at its source by appealing to the Mancunian newly-weds.

The world food supply is in a precarious state. It is increasing arithmetically, and irregularly, at approximately 1 per cent per year, while the human population increases geometrically at 1·8 per cent. India, despite a population density only one-half that of the United Kingdom, is dependent on North American surpluses for one-third of her food, but the United States has expanded its own population from 143 million to 200 million since V.J. Day. She has already warned of her declining capacity to assist India in the future. The World Health Organisation recommends 2·5 acres as the minimal area required per person for food and fibre production. We have only 0·8 of an acre each in England and Wales of which only 0·6 is usable. In consequence, England and Wales import 40 per cent of their food, for which New Zealand farmers are perennially grateful.

The congestion in high-density urban areas breeds psychological stresses; 'pathological togetherness', 'flat neurosis' and mental pollution. The incidence of physical and mental illness rises floor by floor in multi-storey units. One Local Authority in Staffordshire requires prospective flat-dwellers to have a medical examination to eliminate potential fall-outs. If we seek temporary respite from urban smog the major trunk and secondary roads in England provide only 11·8 yards per vehicle.

But turning to some of the medical aspects. Obstretrics is one game at which practice does not make perfect. A woman having her sixth child faces six times the maternal mortality of the second confinement and the sixth child is exposed to twice the risk of perinatal death compared with the second born.

And what of the British tax-payer? The Welfare State has made pregnancy a community affair. Every year £250 million must be found to provide for the care of pregnant women and their progeny. The annual expenditure on maternity services is £21 million in maternity benefits and £36 million in maternity allowances paid to patients, while family allowances now account for £190 million. There is the added burden of the large 'problem' family. The Sociology Department of York University estimates that these families cost the tax-payer £50–£200 per week.

The size of family which ensures a zero rate of population growth is 2·2, that is, each couple can reproduce their two selves, with every fifth couple, or so, having a third but not a fourth child to make up for those who have one or none. Thus, the traditional desire to have children of both sexes must, regrettably, be denied to some. The present global rate of increase of population by 1·8 per cent per annum is arising from an average family size of 3·5. One child less per family and the world would be within sight of demographic parity. Although improved and possibly new methods of contraception will doubtless emerge, existing techniques are sufficiently effective to lower the family size to the level of 2·2. A normally fertile couple takes on average four months to conceive, giving a conception rate of 300 per 100 woman years of exposure. This can be reduced by oral contraceptive to 0·1, by intra-uterine contraceptive devices to 4, by diaphragms and sheaths to 10, by the rhythm method to 24 (calendar), and 18 (temperature) per 100 woman years of exposure. Despite the efficiency of modern contraceptive methods 50 per cent of women do not become strongly motivated towards family limitation until they have 3 children, rising to 90 per cent when they have 6 children. Recent surveys in London showed that in social classes 1 and 2, 20 per cent of pregnancies were unplanned, in the lower strata 60 per cent, and 70 per cent of those with unplanned pregnancies had never practised any efficient form of contraception. Whereas 33 per cent of Australasian women now take the pill and 25 per cent of American women, only 10 per cent do so in the United Kingdom and the world-wide average is 2·5 per cent. To paraphrase the road safety poster, 'Most accidents are caused by people', we might say that 'Most people are caused by accidents'.

Even when some form of family planning is used summation of the decisions of individual couples regarding the size of their family, plus their unplanned conceptions, does not add up to good national policy. Governments should give a definite lead. A useful start was made in this country with the Family Planning Act 1967, which empowered and required Local Authorities to provide contraceptive advice and materials. Unfortunately, the Act did not include the two other major branches of the National Health Service, the hospital and general practitioner divisions, under whose aegis the majority of women have their post-natal examinations. This is undoubtedly the most useful time to offer family planning. Unfortunately, the Local Health Authorities seldom handle patients at this critical stage. In addition to adopting family planning as national policy, governments should introduce indirect methods, such as strong economic disincentives to large families and more generous tax allowances for married women who work outside the home. Perhaps the present maternity grants should be replaced by a 'non-maternity bonus' paid conveniently, if not appropriately, each Christmas to every married woman who has not called upon the maternity or gynaecological services during that year.

Although the Family Planning Act 1967 carefully avoided differentiating between married and unmarried, and Hansard showed that this was deliberate policy, one half of the Local Authorities in England and Wales are locked in bitter controversy as to whether or not the unmarried should be given contraceptive advice and appliances. Denmark is much more progressive. Since 1966 any girl between 15 and 18 years of age can demand that any doctor or birth clinic supply her with an effective contraceptive appliance or drug, as can any woman who has had a child or miscarriage. In the first year the birth rate fell by 7·4 per cent. In this country Brook Clinics pioneered by Mrs Helen Brook have been established in many cities and are doing excellent work in making contraceptives available to the unmarried who are at risk. It is wrong to ignore this problem, and it is wrong to withhold contraceptives from those who request them, as the tragedy of an unwanted pregnancy transcends all other considerations. However, the birth of an unwanted child is not the only misuse of sex. There is an obvious need to instruct adolescents in all aspects of sexual behaviour – physiological, psychological, and sociological, as well as in contraceptive methods, so that they will develop a responsible attitude in contrast to the bravado which motivates many of them at present. Since most parents have abdicated from the responsibility of providing sexual education to their adolescent children, the schools must take up the task by default.

Since I accepted the invitation to contribute to this series Pope Paul has published his encyclical, *Humanæ Vitæ*. Initially, I was as disappointed as any of his co-religionists, but on reflection he may have done this world a service by focusing attention on birth control at this time because time is running short if the world is not to face the Four Horsemen of the Apocalypse. The Papal prohibition on contraception will directly influence reproduction amongst the 600 million Roman Catholics, that is one-sixth of the world's population, and by keeping birth control off the agenda of the World Health Organisation it will indirectly affect those developing countries which have applied to the United Nations for help. Whatever the ethical and moral aspects there are but two ways of checking the ability of humans to populate the world beyond its capacity to sustain life. One is to allow the death rate to increase, by destroying all antibiotic factories, immunisation centres, blood banks, and artificial kidney units, and by closing most hospitals. The other is to reduce the birth rate. If we do not use what little time is left to encourage voluntary methods of birth control, desperate measures will become obligatory, probably before the end of this century.

DUNSTAN Mr Francis has accurately, and with masterly summary power, described a situation and prescribed a remedy. I have been asked to comment upon some of the ethical problems to which the widespread practice of birth control gives rise. Now it is a sign of genius in a university department when it can plan ahead of events, for since this discussion was planned the encyclical, *Humanæ Vitæ*, has been published and has plunged the Roman Catholic Church into a controversy from which all its friends must hope it will soon emerge, enlarged in liberty and understanding. The encyclical is not my subject here: I am a Church of England man. We in our church are entirely at one with the Roman Church in our regard for the integrity of marriage and the family, and in affirming the positive duty of responsible parenthood. We differ only about the means by which this end may be achieved. The Roman Church permits some means but not others; the Church of England leaves the choice to the conscientious decision of the husband and wife concerned. That is all. However, in so far as the encyclical is addressed beyond the frontiers of the Roman Church, 'to all men of goodwill', I accept it as addressed also to me. But then I must show myself to be a man of goodwill in my reply to it – and so surely must we all in this discussion, for it is only with goodwill that the force of reason can be brought to bear. And our subject now is what part has reason to play in that most unreasonable of all human pursuits, the sexual expression of human love? This is not simply a debating paradox; it is the critical question for us here.

The act of sexual love is a human act. This is primary; it has in it an animal ingredient in that it derives its force, and one of its ends or consequences, from those biological drives which we share with many other members of the animal kingdom. It is nevertheless a human act, because we have invested it with characteristics which are not found within the animal kingdom, but which are peculiarly our own. We recognise that this act yields its full potential only when it is part of an exclusive and continuous one-to-one relationship between man and woman, and when that relationship is one of affection and love. We have built it into the emotional life of men and women, and we have submitted it to their reasoned moral judgement and control. We have learned that its biological purpose or consequence is not the only one of which it is capable. It is, therefore, an essentially spontaneous act, a relationship into which the spouses can will themselves with joyful abandon. We cannot lose this spontaneity without losing something of its humanity. And yet reason must come in, as the servant of the goodwill and fundamental human respect which the spouses owe to each other and to the biological consequence of their union – the children which they beget. Reason, like spontaneity, is an attribute of humanity. We can be as inhuman in denying reason, as in denying the spontaneity of love.

It was the exercise of reason which gave us the knowledge upon which birth control is grounded: the understanding of the biological process; the understanding of the two purposes or functions of marital love, the one unitive, the other procreative; the understanding that, while every act of union ought to serve the unitive end, not every act must serve the procreative end; the understanding of how, on any given occasion, we may separate the two. All this we owe to reason, to other people's reason first of all, but which we share as the common possession of the human race. The response to this benefit must surely be a reasoned one: the making of reasoned choices in those fields where choices are open to us, and the facing reasonably of the consequences of our actions and of our common corporate possession of this knowledge. This is precisely what we call ethics. It is part of our humanity to face some of the ethical problems to which the widespread practice of birth control gives rise.

My purpose, therefore, is neither to encourage the practice of birth control nor to dissuade from it, but rather to accept as a fact that the practice is widespread and to consider some of the ethical problems that arise. How widespread it is a simple pair of figures will tell us. We take startled glances at countries like Africa, Asia, and Latin America, where the proportion of the population under the age of fifteen is upwards of 40 per cent, compared with our present figure in England and Wales of about 23 or 24 per cent. But here in England and Wales in 1871, our under-fifteens numbered

36·5 per cent, because our reproductive habits then had hardly yet begun to change, whereas medical science was already keeping many more babies alive. We went through a process a century ago, which these other countries with a rapid population growth are passing through now, though they have greater numbers involved and less wealth and industrial potential to sustain the growth. To-day we all share potentially the same benefits from medical science in prolonging life. However unevenly we share them is not, at present, to the point. Yet because of very widespread family planning, our population here is more or less under control, while theirs without it is not.

What follows ethically from this? Assuming that we admit any relevant obligation towards countries with over-rapid population growth, one duty must be to help them secure something like the balance of population growth with economic resources which has been achieved elsewhere. But how is this to be done? If the facts of our own history are any guide, it is not simply by campaigning for more birth control there. England is not relatively wealthy because it has limited its population – the case is precisely the reverse. England was able to limit its population because of its relative wealth, because its industrial and economic development enabled it to offer human possibilities to children, if there were not too many of them. I wrote about this some years ago in a book called *The Family is not Broken*,[1] and I don't think I can improve very much now on what I said then:

> People do not undertake the discipline, even the simplest, involved in family planning until they have some awareness of the child as a person in himself; as one who is to be loved and cared for as himself; one for whom certain goals and opportunities are desirable for his own real or supposed good. These goals and opportunities must be attainable. They must be seen to be within reach; and then the family will deny itself in various ways, alter its pattern of living where necessary, in order to reach them. So it is that family planning follows in the wake of education and industrialisation together: education, enlarging the mind's apprehension of life and (if it be true education) of the value of personality and, at the same time, giving the skills, the means, by which to attain the goals and opportunities in the wealthier society which industry creates.

[1] G. R. Dunstan, *The Family is not Broken* (SCM Press, 1962, p.27).

The worst enemy of responsible parenthood is fatalism, despair, and this is what we have first to conquer.

Thus my prescription for helping to solve the population problem today is an oblique one, which subordinates all economic, social and political action to respect for the family unit, the married couple, and the integrity of their own marital relationship. Of course, there must be massive economic intervention and change, with profound social and political consequences. But this will succeed precisely as and when it wins a response, wins co-operation, wins the aid of reason to goodwill in the husbands and wives vitally concerned. The population problem is a human problem, and its solution must be found in human terms, in respect for the total humanity of the persons involved. This requires us not to treat men and women as objects to be manipulated by economic, or fiscal, or political means – by bribing, or taxing, or compelling them to follow a population policy laid down on the assumption that because they are hungry and poor they are passive and can be made to conform.

Man is properly a man when he is active, an agent, not passive. This statement I would support with two types of argument. First, an argument from the process of evolution itself. Man is himself part of nature, of the evolving created order. Of all creatures in that order man has gone furthest, so far as we know, in acquiring power over nature and in using it not only to subdue his environment to his own ends, but also to advance his own evolutionary development. This is a proud claim but a true one and therefore one to be made with proper humility. The conscious and deliberate control of the process of reproduction is one means of this development. Now, I grant that there is a solidarity in human affairs which enables some men to do things on behalf of other men, and for their supposed good, and for that of 'society'. But one aspect of man's humanity is his insistence that there are limits to what may be properly done for other men, or rather to them, without their free co-operation and consent. This insistence is particularly strong in protecting the essential human relationship of marriage and its consummation. The necessity of respecting man's agency is surely recognised by every practitioner in medicine, or in education, or in social work, in the psychology of the dependent patient, or pupil, or client, and the problem of getting him on or well. Multiply this on a world scale and you see the point of my contention: we have first to fight apathy and despair and win co-operation.

My second argument is simply a theological one. The Hebrew and Christian tradition, stemming from the myth or symbolic story in Genesis, sets man firmly in the creative order, himself a creature of God. Yet it speaks also of a dominion or lordship given to man by God, and for which man is responsible to God. In speaking of man made in the image of God, it asserts his capacity for response and for relationship, and supremely for relationship with God. And it asserts that these relationships, which are man's chief characteristic, are themselves sacred in the sense that their violation is a violation of what is characteristically human about man. It is significant, perhaps, that natural and medical science, by which this dominion over nature has been extended, has progressed most in a civilisation permeated by this Jewish and Christian doctrine of creation and of man.

So, in this context, man and wife together are to be respected as joint agents in the transmission of life and in the evolution of society; and their own self-respect, essential to this agency, has to be won. And because, after due preparation, the final training in responsibility comes with taking it, the critical decisions in family planning must be left to the reason and consciences of the spouses themselves.

I have woven a rather complex argument with the interplay of personal decisions and social consequences – of the domestic approach to parenthood and the world's concern with population. The reason for this complexity is that I have to make two ethical refusals. I refuse to regard family planning as primarily an instrument of population policy. I see it primarily as a function of the integrity of the marriage, something required by the mutual respect or love of husband and wife, and by their common respect or love for their children. But secondly I have to refuse to isolate their marital and family unit from the society in which they are part. I have to affirm their duty to give responsible thought to society and its needs, as I have to affirm the duty of the State, the Church, and of all outside agencies to respect their integrity in their marriage. I have not gone very far in pursuing other ethical consequences, and the reason for this is not difficult to see. It is that an assessment of ethical consequences must take full account of social consequences; and these are hard enough to trace and analyse after the event – he would be a rash man now who would predict them, especially without adequate demographic and sociological training. Let me cite one simple example concerning the age structure of the population and some of its consequences.

What happens to a country, like our own or like Japan, when families with a large number of surviving children are quickly replaced by small families? It follows that a generation or two later there will be what is loosely called 'a problem of old people' in that country, some with no relatives at all, some with none near them, and altogether forming a statistically disproportionate section of the population. Then equally suddenly – as happened here immediately after World War II, and to some extent before it – people begin to marry earlier, more people marry and many have rather larger families than their parents had, and all this in a short span of years. This creates another bulge – one at the bottom of the pyramid as well as one at the top. This produces what is called a high dependency differential, with a small working group in the middle having to produce wealth and services enough for large dependent groups of children and old people at either end. The social and economic consequences of this are far-reaching. They lead, among other things, to the acceptance of a high number of immigrants from overseas, as in all the industrialised countries of Western Europe now. This in turn creates more problems, and all with their own ethical demands, some of which we are facing. This does not mean that the multitude of personal decisions which produce smaller or larger families were wrong. It means only that their consequences follow for long afterwards, and a humane society is one which will use all its corporate wisdom and resources to deal with them. This I cite as one simple example of the complexity of the social consequence of individual decisions and of the necessity for ethical consideration of them one by one as they come, and indeed, altogether in their total complexity. We should also be wise, when prediction is possible, to give them preliminary thought before they arise: too many of our ethical problems are with us simply for lack of adequate forethought and forward planning.

Lord Cohen then invited questions from the audience.

C. TAYLOR It is inevitable that, in this matter, the doctor's own moral posture is of some influence when he is consulted, particularly by the unmarried, for contraceptive advice, and this gives rise to certain problems. Particularly in Liverpool, quite a large number of the student population are unfortunately denied easy access to birth control advice. In the light of the very challenging statement by Mr Francis, in which he says that he considers that all coitus without efficient contraception, extra-marital, non-marital, and in marriage after the birth of three children, irresponsible, I would ask the question of the platform, is, therefore, the doctor's behaviour in this context also immoral? Mr Francis, is your behaviour irresponsible, my Lord Chairman, is your behaviour unethical, Professor Dunstan, is your behaviour immoral? A corollary to this dilemma (and it is a dilemma which faces many doctors, particularly in general practice where rightly patients feel they have the most confidential and the easiest sort of access) is when a doctor is consulted, or a clinic is consulted, by patients who have already been refused advice, by their general practitioner. One insists, if oral contraception is advised, that this is a chemical that it is only right and proper that the patient's own doctor should know is being taken. There are certain side effects, and it is quite wrong, particularly in emergencies, that someone responsible for health should not know of this particular form of chemical treatment. Also what is the situation when the patient, who is only consulting you and is not your regular patient, insists that they do not wish their own general practitioner to be informed? Should you then refuse to prescribe an oral contraceptive, or should you prescribe what is asked for, so long as the patient is aware of the risks involved?

FRANCIS I am displeased that all three medical officers of the student medical service of this University of Liverpool refuse to provide students with any form of contraceptive appliance, or with the pill. Approximately two per cent of female university students drop out each year because of pregnancy. Tax-payers are forced to invest a thousand pounds per student each year. I have made students welcome in my consulting rooms for some time because I feel that it is wasteful economically, and from the viewpoint of the student's own career, to refuse contraceptive assistance. These students are showing some degree of responsibility for their actions by asking for assistance. The ones who are irresponsible are those who do not seek help. This is one situation where one cannot observe all of the medical niceties of the past. I agree with the questioner that there is a contraceptive problem among the student population in this city and I think that a body such as the Senate of the University should made a broad statement of policy for the guidance of the staff of the Student Medical Service.

DUNSTAN I would distinguish between a principle and the means by which it is commended or upheld. And with regard to the means, I would distinguish between the personal or professional judgement given by an individual person in a given situation and the public policy which forms the background against which those decisions and those judgements are made. For myself, I wish to uphold the principle that the only proper context for sexual union is marriage. How then is this principle to be commended or upheld? First the doctor in his professional conversation with the patient has to make up his mind (if he accepts this principle) whether the giving or withholding of contraceptive facilities is going to commend it to the patient or not: whether he or she will be fortified or won over to this position, or not. The doctor has to make his own judgement of the probabilities. On the matter of public policy lying behind this, I think a policy of refusal of contraceptive advice to the unmarried cannot now be said to be an effective, or expedient, or even a just method of upholding the principle which I wish to see upheld. A just and effective public policy must now allow for both those personal and professional judgements to be taken.

M. J. BATESON I should like to ask Mr Francis if he envisages that the introduction of the pill as well as providing contraception will help sublimate maternal instinct which still causes intelligent and well-educated women to pour the energies of the best years of their lives into child rearing.

FRANCIS I feel that it is necessary to substitute a real interest outside the home for what has previously taken up so many years of women's lives. Regarding 'maternal instinct' I shall shock most of you by saying that I have come to the conclusion that for the majority of women 'maternal instinct' is an anachronistic euphemism for female libido. Throughout twenty years in full-time hospital appointments I did not realise the inhibiting effect of nurses and students upon patients at the post-natal examination. In the privacy of my consulting room I am amazed at the frequency with which patients state that there must be something wrong with their maternal instinct because they do not like the baby. They would not do it any harm, they look after it well, they feed and clothe it, and if necessary defend it, but they would prefer to return to their pre-pregnancy status. The first reaction of any woman to pregnancy is that she wishes to be unpregnant. She wants to be pregnant at some more convenient time in the future, even next month, but not now. Maternal instinct is something which needs investigating. I agree that if you are to ask people to restrict their families to two children you must provide them with a career outside the home to which to devote their interest, energy and time.

J. H. CLIFFORD I feel that there was one point at which the speakers seemed to be in conflict. Professor Dunstan rather glossed over Mr Francis's 1·8 per cent annual increase of our population – or the doubling of the population in approximately thirty years. He did, however, stress a point which I know from public health work is engaging many people's attention as a serious problem, namely that of the ageing population, and he pointed out that this was one of the consequences of diminishing birth rates. I wonder if both speakers could give their opinions as to how this is to be reconciled.

DUNSTAN On the statistical level I am not competent to discuss this at any depth because I have not the figures at my fingertips. So far as my reading and listening on the BBC has informed me there is not a serious problem of rapid population growth in this country. There is a serious problem of the distribution of the density of our population and I should not wish to see it multiply at a higher rate than it is at present. But I do not think we have grounds for serious alarm: though indeed I may be mistaken about this. I do remember that the great predictions of the thirties about the decline of population in this country, and indeed throughout Western Europe, were quite markedly and quickly falsified.

Long before the Population Commission, which was set up to investigate, had reported its findings the situation had altered itself. There is an extraordinary self-regulating mechanism in a society like ours with so many inter-related factors, so that I can well believe that the tendency of the crude birth rate of the last two years may be initiating a phase of smaller families. I am a little alarmed at the continuing decline in the age of marriage. We appear to be going back to that system of child marriage from which large tracts of the Earth are crying out to be delivered, and child marriage does produce a population increase by shortening the gap between the generations, as well as creating problems for the spouses themselves and for their families. But again, this is not an irreversible trend, and I should not like to predict rapidly approaching disaster for this country. As for the ageing population, I think we have yet to reach the peak of this superabundance of ageing people. It may come, though I'm not certain, in the 1980s, but it will certainly pass. It was a product of the large families of three to four generations ago, followed by the immediately sharply reduced families of the first-war years and the twenties; but this will phase itself out. I mentioned the point to illustrate that a rapid, sudden, and widespread change of family habits produces consequences for a long time afterwards – and that each of these consequences in its turn, and the totality of them together, raises ethical questions because further problems are created which we have to tackle.

FRANCIS First a correction: the English population is increasing at 0·8 per cent per year, the world population at 1·8 per cent. Changes in population are serious matters, for changes gain momentum and are difficult to arrest. An increase in the birth rate of a community makes its first impact on the obstetric services, then the elementary schools, followed by secondary schools, universities, and industry. For some years this country has been embarrassed by having more children than places in primary schools. It costs the tax-payer £250 million to add 800,000 children to the British population each year, approximately £300 per conception. If annual births were reduced to parity with annual deaths, viz. 500,000, £100 million could be diverted to the senior citizens.

It is the middle-aged section of the community which supports the young and the old. A drastic reduction in the birth rate would cause a narrow waist to move through the various age strata. However, it would occur but once. A desirable population structure is the shape of Cleopatra's needle as opposed to both the pyramid and the egg-timer. With 500,000 births per annum we would achieve a Cleopatra-needle age distribution and we would not face calamitous years when a narrow-waist stratum reached middle-age.

A. SPEAKMAN From what Mr Francis has said, I feel that he visualises a situation where the State will have to pass laws limiting the number of children people can have, whether married or unmarried. Now would he like to say quite clearly to what extent he is going to allow the State to interfere between his clinical judgement and his patient?

FRANCIS I do not think that this would necessarily arise. What we do need is implementation of the Family Planning Act to make it true national policy, together with fairly liberal legislation covering tubal ligation and vasotomy. We could eliminate the surplus one-third of a million pregnancies each year. If that were not sufficient there could be some further liberalisation of the Abortion Law, but I do not think that anyone should come between me and the patient and instruct the patient, 'you are pregnant for the fourth time, you are therefore directed to enter a gynaecological unit and you must permit the pregnancy to be terminated.'

SPEAKMAN I must apologise for the misunderstanding then, but your whole argument seems to be towards the conclusion that this situation is inevitable unless something is done; and what you are assuming, quite wrongly I think, is first of all that maternal instincts are just an expression of female libido – I think you've got it the wrong way round – and secondly that there would never be, no matter how great the population, any reversal of the instinct of man to procreate himself. Now I want you again to answer the question. In the situation which I think we have envisaged, the State would have to interfere with the free choice of a person. If that person wanted to continue having children, and the State said, 'No, your doctor must make it impossible for you to do so,' would you allow that to happen?

FRANCIS I do not think that this is at all necessary and I certainly would not be a party to this. Most governments have policies which encourage people to have larger families. For instance, they do not give any allowance for the first child, but 18s. for the second child and £1 for the third, plus income tax allowances for all progeny. Such policies could be reversed by giving taxation advantages to people who have one or two children, allowances ceasing with the third child with punitive taxation for those with more than four children.

DUNSTAN I think this debate needs to be kept above questions which are more domestic than general. It is important to do so because here we are touching a very important point of social ethics and public policy, namely the question of how far we want direct intervention by Act of Parliament both into the realm of married life and into professional practice. I want to keep them as far away from both as possible. Clearly in the matter before us family allowances are a hangover from a demographic past. They were introduced as a measure of population policy precisely during that time of rapid narrowing of families in the twenties and thirties of which I spoke just now. And this is why they continue unchanged.

Now I agree that the population of a country and the age composition of that population must be a matter of concern to its government. It would be irresponsible of any government to ignore it. Yet in making the policies which are going to express that concern there are certain principles which any government today must respect, as well as political advantages upon which it must calculate. If we are going to discuss a population policy for this country it can be done perfectly well within the terms dictated by these two considerations. Certainly when we examine critically and rationally the whole wages structure, salary structure and systems of remuneration and national insurance, the incentive of family allowances, as now made, could very well fall away – once it becomes politically possible to remove them. I, however, believe that, given a society such as ours, with vast potential, both economic and social, and given a population becoming steadily more educated, we hope, and in some ways, also, more responsible, we can in fact rely upon the interplay of reasonable decisions with the help of persuasive policies to settle this, without compulsion and without the intervention of laws that are going to impinge upon family life or professional practice.

SYLVIA BENSON I am an ex-SRN, so I've seen a bit of life. I should just like to make one or two observations. Six years ago I went to nurse outside Chicago for a couple of years and when I first went there I was shocked; practically every woman was sterilised after her fourth baby. But now I'm not sure that they were wrong. Don't you think we need a different standard of morality? We must separate sex and conception. I mean we must teach young people that whatever they do sexually that's their own affair; it's entirely between their conscience and God so long as they keep their bodies clean and avoid VD. But we must teach that to bring an unwanted, unloved, unwelcome, unhoused baby into the world is a wicked, wicked thing.

FRANCIS I agree completely with what you have said: the ultimate tragedy is the production of an illegitimate child. The illegitimate births in this country have not only doubled in the past decade but all strata of society are now equally involved. There was a time when illegitimate births were almost confined to the lower social strata.

BARNETT Dr Speakman really asked the question that I am about to level again. It is concerning this question of compulsion which to me touches upon the fundamental moral issue. Both speakers seem essentially in agreement, except that Professor Dunstan did not think the problem of overpopulation was quite upon us, but Mr Francis did, and he presented it very competently and almost terrifyingly. But I would like Professor Dunstan to accept that the position could be upon us and in the light of that to answer the question. I would ask both speakers, therefore: When attempts to influence people have failed, are they in favour of compulsion? There are people who say family allowance be damned, and whatever incentive you give me be damned, I'm going to have ten children. Would the speakers expect there then to be State interference?

FRANCIS As with so many things in this world there comes a time when one has to give in, even though forecasts of the results of population explosions are terrifying. I believe that we have only ten to fifteen years in which to halt the present increase in world population and not more than twenty-five to thirty years in this country. However, there comes a time when there is direct conflict between human liberty and demography. Finally one has to give in and let people have their pregnancies rather than to terminate them by government decree. I would plead that we use what little time is left to reduce the birth rate voluntarily, to avoid having to adopt such measures as abortion on demand. Japan is currently terminating over one million of two and a half million conceptions per annum and Hungary is aborting over 60 per cent of all conceptions. There is no compulsion in either country. Abortion is merely available on demand. I would anticipate that legalising abortion 'on demand' in this country would lead to an equally high percentage of terminated pregnancies.

DUNSTAN I, in general, don't dissent from that view. I should like to distinguish three elements in the problem which I think are rather confused. There is, one, the world population problem, with which I share the alarm of anyone. There is secondly the population growth of this country, about which I am not alarmed, because I think the hypothetical possibility outlined won't happen. There are enough mechanisms regulating things from within to make the tide turn before anything like a frightening population problem, given the present social structure, will come about, in this country. Thirdly, there is the area of personal, individual decision, of the sort that might result in a person insisting on having ten children. Now I refuse in principle any compulsion in this matter. I do not wish to see compulsion exerted upon doctors and other medical persons, which interfere with their professional code of ethics. I do not wish to see the encouragement of large-scale abortion by any means at all in this country. These strong-arm methods, drastic methods, of compulsion or of surgery, will in the long run tend to dehumanise; my fundamental belief is that the only solution to this problem is to be found in a higher sense of humanity and respect for it, not in a lower. If in the end we die, well then we die. It is more human to die than to live in a sub-human way.

COHEN Though there has been a different point of view expressed by the speakers, I think ultimately they reached the same conclusion; that any control of a population explosion must be on a voluntary basis. Mr Francis expressed his credo very clearly in his belief that coitus without efficient contraception is irresponsible and anti-social in all pre-marital and extra-marital affairs, and after the birth of the third child within marriage. Then he painted, as a questioner pointed out, a grave and indeed terrifying picture of a starving, thirsty and overcrowded population. It would be difficult for me to insist that health education of any kind yielded very worthwhile results. Hitherto certainly it has not done so, except in those fields in which the contribution by the individual is so small that it hardly matters, as, for example, in immunisation and mass radiology. But the view which Mr Francis expressed is certainly one which has to be taken into account and, as he rightly says, if there is an increase in birth rate over a death rate, then sooner or later some measure of control may well have to be introduced. But I suspect that it will be introduced from within the community and not imposed by governmental edict.

Professor Dunstan has dealt with the ethical problems, which he approaches by the light of reason. His very significant point that marital love is not simply procreative, but also unitive, is, of course, of prime importance. And then he insists that it is reason which determines how these shall be separated. Having accepted that the practice of birth control is widespread, he then maintains, with rather different emphasis from Mr Francis, that it is important to subordinate the social, economic and political consequences of an increased birth rate, to respect for the family unit and its integrity. He refuses to regard family planning as primarily an instrument of population policy, though he believes it is important that individuals should have some regard for the needs of society and the State.

IV HUMAN GUINEA-PIGS

LORD PLATT

PLATT I should like to put before you illustrations of certain circumstances in which modern medicine has revealed ethical problems which require a solution. By no means all these are new, but modern drugs are much more potent, both for good and for ill, than old ones and modern operations are much more miraculous, for good or ill, than old-fashioned ones, which were tentative and exploratory. So new problems have arisen, not only in the field of therapy – that is the treatment of the patient – but also in the field of public health, where we are sometimes up against the decision as to whether we should urge a very large number of the population to have some kind of inoculation, the dangers of which are not fully known. Such an experiment is not so much for the benefit of the individual patient (because the chances of the individual getting poliomyelitis are small) but for the benefit of the population at large. There are also areas in which we come rather unexpectedly and abruptly into the field of politics, and last, but not least, there is the almost new field of organ transplantation.

First of all there is the situation in which we are sincerely trying to treat the patient, and not really to do anything else, but we may be trying a new remedy. It may only be a minor modification of what has gone before, and nobody's very frightened by it, and one does not have to say to the patient: 'You know, this particular modification of this drug has not been used before.' A doctor always has to use his own judgement as to how much alarm he should cause a patient. You might, for instance, be treating migraine headaches with a new remedy. It is up to you as a responsible doctor to assure yourself by various means that the appropriate tests have been done, and now the Safety in Drugs Committee should ensure that the manufacturers have taken every reasonable precaution to test the drug in animal experiments, and often, on volunteers in their own departments. So assuming that you are satisfied with tests made, then you have a right to test out the new drug, without, so to speak, advertising to the patient that this is an experiment. Very often the gain is marginal, and you may have to do a carefully controlled experiment to make sure that results are really meaning something, and are not simply due to your own enthusiasm, which you may pass on to the patient. So you may have to devise a controlled experiment, in which some people are given the drug, and others are not, and they don't know who is having the drug, so their own bias is laid aside, and they're not tempted to think they are better on the new drug. Or you may have to do a controlled experiment, not with one treatment against another, but with one treatment against a control, a harmless tablet, which has no effect whatever, and contains only a little sugar, or something of that kind. This is called a placebo. Now, it is my view – and it is open to discussion – that controlled experiments of this kind should never be done without the patient's co-operation, even if the illness is not dangerous, and your remedy is probably not dangerous, and your placebo is certainly harmless. It is my view that this kind of experiment should not bc done without the patient's consent if only because you are a doctor, and you would be deceiving a patient. This is against the code of medical ethics. I think it is bad to bring up students to think that they can deceive patients. It's perfectly easy to get the collaboration of intelligent patients who realise that one fortnight they're going to have treatment, another fortnight they're not, and they're not going to know which it is, and they're going to tell you at the end which they think it is. But, of course, now and then one of the drugs you're going to test is going to turn out to have potential dangers. The case of thalidomide is still *sub judice*, and one must not make statements entirely attibuting certain effects to a certain drug, but this at least was a very disturbing situation – when it appeared that the administration of this drug early in pregnancy was likely to be followed by an increased liability to deformity amongst the babies that were born. I mention it because my own view is that you can never say, however carefully you test a drug, that 'this will never happen again'. There are species differences. If you test this, or some other drug on pregnant animals, you will find that in one species, which might be the rabbit, nothing untoward happens at all, but if you try it on a rat or a guinea-pig something would happen that would have put you on your guard.

I see no way of finding this out in advance, unless every drug is going to be tested for years with almost every animal you can think of, in which case the benefits of the new drugs would be delayed by many years. This pinpoints the importance of the early warning system which was introduced by the Royal College of General Practitioners, and is now taken up by the Safety in Drugs Committee, in which doctors are invited to send in details of any untoward circumstance in a patient that might possibly be due to some drug that they were having. This may happen only once in thousands of times. There may be one doctor who practises in Henley and has a patient with severe anaemia, and he has almost forgotten he prescribed the drug: another doctor in Glasgow had such a patient, another one in Paris had such a patient, and the things are never connected, unless all doctors are invited to say, 'This is a mysterious anaemia; this patient has been having the following drugs,' and other doctors do the same.

However, our subject is human experiment, and I am only telling you that it can never be entirely safe, but as long as you are completely on the side of the patient, I would say that you are on sound ground ethically. You try to do your best: you are weighing up the possible dangers against the possible benefits. You are seeking a conclusion which of course occasionally may turn out to be the wrong one.

However, we may not only be testing out drugs. We may be testing operations, or we may be trying out something as simple as whether you keep patients at home or send them into hospital, but the ethical problem is very largely the same. There are ways by which the heart, if it suddenly stops, can be restarted with such complete success that the patient eventually goes back to work, and there are other times in which the heart goes into a dangerous state of irregularity which can be put back to normal quite simply by modern apparatus. These are risks that may happen when a person has a coronary attack. If he is in hospital, monitored by modern apparatus, there will be a team ready to act if something suddenly goes wrong. So you would say, well then surely all the coronary patients should be sent into hospital where they can have these facilities, and presumably it is unethical to keep such patients at home. But the counter observation has been made that most patients with coronary disease die within a few hours, if they are going to die at all. And if you move them into hospital, quite a large number of them die in the ambulance or within an hour of admission to hospital, and so we must ask, are the benefits of immediate resuscitation and monitoring greater than those of leaving the patient at home? This is a very tricky subject in medical ethics. The only way of really settling this is a statistical trial in which you say at random, patients A, C, D and F will go into hospital; patients B, E and G will stay at home. You will then get a large number of people telling you that this is an unethical thing, that the hospital has all this apparatus which you are denying to patients. We have, in fact, an investigation of this kind going on and it transpires that, in the early stages, the patients who stay at home do rather better than those who go into hospital! So you see if your immediate reaction was that this was an unethical experiment, you would have to do a little rethinking. I need hardly say that all kinds of safeguards were put into this, in the sense that if there were some compelling reason – even the wish of the patient, which is a very compelling reason – why this patient should go into hospital and not stay at home, or vice versa, then this overruled the whole experiment and the patient was not included at all. In other words, if you are going to do this kind of controlled experiment, your conscience must be quite clear that you do not know which is going to turn out to be the better – otherwise you shouldn't do the experiments.

When we come to the subject of investigation rather than treatment, we are on a good deal more delicate ground, but again we are fairly safe as long as we are doing an investigation because we think it will throw light on a particular patient's illness. This patient is very seriously ill, not perhaps going to die next week or two, but with not more than a few months to live if some important cardiac operation is not performed. But is it going to be the right operation? Is it going to do him any good? You are, I think, entitled to experiment if you are reasonably sure that the risk is small and that the benefit may be considerable. And, I would say again, that as you are doing it for the patient's sake you need not explain that every step is experimental. On the other hand I think the real area for criticism is where experiments are done, not for the benefit of the patient, but in order to contribute to the sum total of medical knowledge with a view that some day when we understand more about a particular disease, this may eventually benefit somebody else. In this case I hold quite strongly that these kind of investigations must go on. There could be no rule which says: 'No you must never do an investigation unless it is absolutely for the benefit of the patient himself.' But I would hold equally strongly that you must have a willing collaborator, and you must explain to the patient what is involved and that perhaps there is a slight risk to be incurred in this kind of experiment; that you're going to put them to some trouble and inconvenience, and that you want them to stay in hospital perhaps a week longer than would otherwise be necessary, but this is going to be important for the progress of medical science. You can easily influence the majority of patients, and the minority you cannot influence at all, so you might as well save your breath. But, to draw a moral from this, you must be fairly sure that the patient really is a willing collaborator, and that nothing you say to the patient relieves you personally of the responsibility of saying to yourself, 'Is this a justifiable experiment?' This is a dividing line that is difficult to define and one where there has been most criticism. And experiments have unquestionably been done of which I'm sure I would not personally approve.

I am now going to outline a few other situations. I said we touch on politics at times. Take driving and alcohol for instance. Careful experiment has shown that if you have around 20 mg of alcohol in your blood you are in fact ever so slightly less likely to have an accident than if you have none at all. Now this may be meaningless, because of how difficult it is to interpret statistics. This could mean that when you are tired, just one glass of sherry does pick you up a bit and you are a better driver. Or it could mean that there is a hard core of frightfully bad drivers – elderly, incompetent, and so on – who never touch alcohol at all and that you have eliminated them by taking only those with 20 mg of alcohol. They don't drive any better; they just drive better than the average driver who never drinks at all. But be that as it may, when you get to the 40 to 50 mg level, the accident rate increases and from then onwards increases enormously so that by 80 mg the accident rate has about doubled and by 110 to 120 mg it is going up sky-high. So this becomes a political decision really. We give the legislators the information, but it is for them to take the political decision: At what level of alcohol in the blood does it become an offence against society to be in charge of a motor-car?

Another political decision comes in with cigarette smoking, which it is estimated now kills about 50,000 people annually in this country. Yet advertisements for cigarettes still appear in nearly every journal.

Then finally we come to dialysis and transplantation for kidney disease, which raises its own very difficult problems because it does raise the question not only of the patient but also of the donor. In earlier kidney transplantations the donor was living, and was usually a close relative, willing to give up a kidney in order that somebody else might benefit from it. This is an ethical problem which is also a statistical problem. I might be willing to give a kidney (if mine are any use) for somebody close to me if I thought he or she had a 90 to 95 per cent chance of recovering as a result of this operation, and was a youngish person. If, though, the chance of him or her making a decent recovery were 3 or 5 per cent I might think very differently about it according to the statistical results. But here we are shooting at a moving target, because unless we go ahead with this kind of thing, the statistical results will never improve, and, as everybody concerned in renal transplantations knows, the results today, the chances of living two, three, four, or five years after a kidney transplant, are very much greater than they were only five years ago.

Finally, the cardiac transplant problem involves the question of a dead donor, so, because organs do not keep indefinitely, we come up against the problem of when is a person dead, knowing full well that people can be dead beyond recovery in their brain yet still can be kept 'alive' so that you can determine the date and time of death by turning off the respirator. These are perhaps the most difficult cases, and certainly the most prominent in the public mind.

The audience then put questions to Lord Platt.

H. J. PRATAP I am a family doctor. In the last twelve months I have had two patients, young mothers with young families, suffering from cancer of the breast. One had surgical treatment, the other had deep X-ray therapy. One died within three months of the treatment, the other within six weeks of the treatment. In neither case did the treatment produce the result expected. On the other side of the scale was an old man of about seventy with cancer of the stomach. The surgeon decided to operate, found he could not do anything and closed him up. The poor man came home and thought he would be better, but he gradually went downhill and died within three months. Another old man of eighty had an enlarged prostate gland. He was operated on, came home, died within six weeks and the wife said he was never the same after the operation. Now I feel that in all these cases there should have been closer co-operation between the family doctor and the surgeon carrying out the treatment, because the family doctor is in the priviledged position of knowing the background of his patients and so could, to a certain extent, influence a surgeon in carrying out the treatment. May I have your view, please?

PLATT I don't honestly think this raises any real ethical problem. Whereas most of us nowadays in the hospital world are conscious of the importance of the extra knowledge that a general practitioner can have of his patients, which in some cases is very important indeed, I would doubt whether, in any of these particular cases, the general practitioner could have predicted the outcome. If he could, he should not have sent them to a surgeon, surely.

N. S. BARNETT I should like to ask Professor Platt about the application of what he understands by morality.

PLATT If I may quote a philosopher, 'Morality is a matter to some extent of rules, right rules. And which are the right rules? Well, the rules that are justified by the right use of practical reason.' And he adds, 'I think that the perception of the right rules is something that comes through living in human relationships and this is why I think it is so important to pay attention to the intuition of experienced ordinary people rather than the prescriptions of the non-humanistic social scientist.' This is one reason why the law is so very unsatisfactory, in that it provides only for extreme cases. They say if you go as far as this then you will be in trouble, but your moral obligations and your own concepts of how these should be interpreted come into action long before that stage is ever reached. For this reason, if for no other, I am very wary, in all discussions on transplant questions and other difficult questions of modern medical ethics, of saying there should be new laws. Public opinion is changing very rapidly, and I am not going to say where I think it will be on this life-and-death matter in five years' time. But I think it might be very different from what it was five years ago, when the subject at issue was keeping people alive. And I suppose if I put myself in the position of the moralist for the moment instead of the physician, and surely they shouldn't be terribly separated, I might say: How mischievous to keep these people alive. If somebody terminates their lives by switching off the machine they are doing what was intended (if we look at it in that way) should happen to them and the mischievous thing has been to keep them alive. Now I'm not saying that I put this forward in every case. Obviously there are all kinds of shades and meanings and so forth but I think one is in at least as strong an ethical position as one is if you say that you must never allow somebody to die so long as you can keep him breathing by a respirator.

COHEN If I might just interpolate one brief comment here; Dr Barnett was trying to establish what determines moral standards; I think that this has been answered and I am sure that others here will be interested in what Lord Esher said in relation to the definition of infamous conduct in a professional respect. The General Medical Council has no code of conduct. It has certain precedents, but every case is judged on its merits and not in relation to a code. There is no law of medical ethics but Lord Esher said that the standard by which a doctor's conduct should be judged is by his professional brethren of good repute and competence. And it seems to me that this is the kind of moral standard at which we are hinting when we speak about how standards might be achieved.

A. N. OTHER I should like to ask a question about consent. Patients' intelligence varies and their knowledge of the normal anatomy and physiology of the human body is sometimes rather scanty. A situation can arise where the patient willingly gives consent to something without having much idea of what he is agreeing to, even though this has been fully explained. What is the moral position here?

PLATT I think this is a point I have already made, but perhaps not strongly enough, and that is, you can never delegate your own final responsibility. To talk patients into anything is one of the worst things. It is almost better, to my mind, to do an experiment that the patient knows nothing about, rather than to talk him into it by virtue of your greater knowledge and personality. I would never have it, in my unit, that because the patient had given consent you can therefore carry on and do what you like. Of course, then it comes back to your own feeling of what your professional responsibilities are. This can be modified by adopting the rule that in an experimental situation of any importance there should be a sort of committee decision. The unit meets and discusses the scope of the investigation and whether it is justifiable, and so on. Some will go further than that and say that at least one member of this committee should be a physician or surgeon completely unconnected with either the patient or the projected piece of research.

S. BENSON Would it not make it easier for doctors if patients, when well and healthy, and in their right mind, gave their doctor some idea of when they wanted to be considered dead? If my brain was severely damaged, I would hope that nobody would try to keep me alive as a cabbage. And I should like it written in my case sheet, just as that I would bequeath my eyes, and my body. And secondly, wouldn't it be kinder and more humane to let long-term prisoners volunteer as guinea-pigs? Surely they would be serving society and making some retribution for their crime.

PLATT In reply to the first question I feel we have to wait for public opinion, and it is my own view that something like this planning will come out of it. The really awful thing is leaving such decisions to relatives at a time when they are suffering bereavement. With regard to prisoners, this is frowned on very much because of the question of consent. Offering inducements like this is very dangerous ground – and the consent is probably not real consent in law, at least it might not be. Is that right, Mr Chairman?

COHEN Well this is so in America. They used to use prisoners quite extensively for human experiments. And a very distinguished Professor of Law, Professor David Daube, of Oxford, spoke in America on some of these ethical problems and he persuaded them that it was absolutely wrong to use prisoners, because whether they thought so or not, the prisoners would certainly be looking for some reward for having volunteered to undergo experiments of this kind. So they have stopped it now in, I think, most states in America.

SANDRA WARD Nobody has mentioned the fact that hospital patients, often without their consent, are used to demonstrate in front of groups of medical students, or student nurses. Are there any comments about this?

PLATT I hold strong views on this. I think demonstration of patients, when the patient is not seen to be a collaborator, is quite barbaric. Some people just don't seem to realise the patient's there, as they lean an elbow on the abdomen, or something of this kind. I have seen a patient wheeled in and out without a single word being spoken to her, and I pretty well wrang the neck of the chap who did it afterwards.

COHEN That was ethical, was it?

PLATT That was! But I do think that a lot of patients don't mind this if you make them a collaborator. If you say, 'Mrs Jones, I want you to tell these young men and women what you were telling me the other day about your illness,' you include her and she is rather pleased about this. This is good, this makes her day – instead of nothing happening to her at all, or going backwards and forwards to the X-ray department. But, of course, if you are going to do this in public, and reveal all the secrets of her illness to an open ward, then this is quite barbaric, and it is time we got away from this, as we all have in the better hospitals.

COHEN But wouldn't you say that you have seldom, if ever, known of a patient objecting if asked beforehand for collaboration?

PLATT A few of them are hesitant; so you explain what you are not going to do, and then they are quite happy about it. They are afraid of being exposed and treated as guinea-pigs in public, and quite reasonably so.

JOHN GOLDSMITH I'm concerned about the ethics of using children for experiment. There are certain drugs, such as vaccines, which by their nature have to be given to children if they are to be assessed. Poliomyelitis vaccine, which of course has been a great boon, is one such drug. Would you discuss the ethics of using a new vaccine such as this for the first time in mentally deficient, rather abnormal children?

PLATT Well, I very much doubt whether this raises a new problem. You are doing this for the benefit of children, and knowing what a horrible disease poliomyelitis is, you are doing it for the benefit of that particular child, though admittedly his chance of getting polio is statistically quite small. But he may do, and so you are trying to protect him from a horrible and lethal disease. This is an experiment in the sense that the vaccine had not been used on this big scale before, but it is not an investigation in the sense of something that is just satisfying your scientific curiosity.

COHEN By way of summing up, may I at the outset say that it seems clear that there are two particular categories one ought to consider. The first is when the human experiment is designed for diagnostic, or therapeutic purposes, and has a specific relevance to the patient on whom the experiment is performed. The second category is where the experiment is undertaken, not for that patient's direct benefit, but to advance knowledge, and this does occasionally mean, as Lord Platt has said, a controlled clinical trial. I would, however, like to stress again what I said earlier, during the discussion, that the fact that there is a *post hoc* justification for an experiment does not justify it. An experiment is ethical, or not, at its inception, and the means cannot justify the end.

If I may speak for the medical profession I would say, and I hope that Lord Platt would agree with me, that only a minority of our professional brethren abuse the privilege and the confidence which is imposed in them. But there is occasionally a lack of public confidence, and that means that we as doctors have to exercise not only *scientia* but also *caritas*. I am delighted that the motto of the Royal College of General Practitioners is *scientia cum caritas* – that is, science combined with compassion. And we of the medical profession must show ourselves to possess that compassion and the highest standards of moral integrity and self-discipline, since it has been said that the final responsibility of coming to a decision as to whether an experiment should be carried out on a human being lies with the doctor himself. I think this is an appropriate moment at which to recall Sir Robert Hutcheson's litany:

> From inability to let well alone, from too much zeal for the new and contempt for what is old, from putting knowledge before wisdom, science before art, cleverness before commonsense, from treating patients as cases, and from making the cure of disease more grievous than the endurance thereof, Good Lord deliver us!

V PSYCHIATRY

D. STAFFORD-CLARK & PETER WINCH

STAFFORD-CLARK In my professional lifetime of endeavour in the field of psychiatry I feel that far too little has been achieved in terms of communication, which is, after all, what we are trying to do. I don't mean by this that people have not been receptive: I mean that they are, as Bernard Shaw pointed out, in receipt of ideas which were out of date fifty years ago. This is despite the fact that various communicators of one sort or another constantly assail them with efforts to bring knowledge up to date.

First of all, what is psychiatry? Well, it can be simply defined as being that part of medicine which is primarily concerned with disorders of thought, feeling and behaviour. In one sense all illness or injury, and indeed all suffering of any kind, involves disorder of feeling and this is one of the reasons why the basic principles of psychiatry are vital to a proper understanding of medicine and surgery as a whole. But the special province of psychiatry is the understanding of those disorders of subjective experience or objective behaviour which are themselves the cause of disability. The nature of the predicament of the patients may be evident to themselves, in which case they are said to have some degree of insight to the nature of their illness; or it may not and they may feel that what is wrong is the world, or their environment, or their body, or that people are against them, in which case they are psychotic in the sense that they are cut off from the rest of the world and the doctor has to reach them before he can in fact either communicate with them or in any way relieve them. All this every doctor must be able to acknowledge, to understand, to diagnose at least in some degree, and also to treat. Psychiatry in fact includes in its concern that most human aspect of human beings, their awareness of themselves and their capacity to communicate with each other. Now you might feel that this was therefore a branch of medicine which was honoured and respected, but in fact this is not so. It is a branch of medicine which is still honoured more in the breach than the observance, and which inspires derision, misconception and fear still as much as any kind of respect or sympathy.

Now I don't think any psychiatrist at this symposium would ask for sympathy for his profession but he would ask for respect for his patients and what he does to them and this brings me straight on to the question of treatment and to misconceptions about it.

Sometimes when I am asked: 'How do you approach a psychiatric patient?' I feel inclined to give the sort of advice which a veterinary surgeon would give to a novice about a horse, namely, 'From in front, visibly and with kindness.' For this reason, a psychiatrist will not permit himself to be introduced as the plumber, or the friend, or somebody's uncle and thereby enter the patient's arena under some subterfuge which may, as far as all others are concerned, be humouring the patient but which in fact is insulting both the patient and the doctor by starting them off on a false basis. Psychiatry, therefore, has to be desperately honest to its patients. It has two ways of treating them: one is by communication and the other is by some physiological intervention. The word intervention has perhaps a slightly alarming ring, but then all treatment in medicine is intervention, we hope mostly for the better, but certainly it is intervention. If you don't intervene, you leave things as you found them, and even masterly inactivity as a policy of treatment is a kind of suspended intervention while you watch to see what happens next. In psychiatry one sometimes does this, but psychiatric treatment can be really approached from the point of view of either the communication angle or the physiological angle, but basically and preferably as a combination of both.

Before I discuss techniques, I would like to point out that the psychiatrist, like any other doctor, faces the problem of what can be done for people from two different angles, one of which he has been very well taught in his medical school and the other of which, until twenty years ago, he was not taught at all, and this is the data with which he has to work. The data are either the neurophysiology of the patient, that is to say the nervous system, and, above all, the brain or the personal and subjective experience of the patient. It was Freud who pointed out that a neurologist or a neurophysiologist could go far into studying the mechanism of conduction, peripheral nerves and communication within the brain.

Today we have knowledge that Freud could not have had fifty

years ago, about the way that the brain works, and we can say with reasonable assurance that the computer analogy, although a far from perfect one, is valid in the sense that the brain is like a computer. It does have a large number of individual nerve cells which are like the transistors in a computer. But some idea of its complexity may be gained by realising that, at the neurophysiological end, there are two or three very important facts which the psychiatrist has to bear in mind when he is thinking about treating the brain physiologically. One is that the brain has 10,000 million cells, which is vastly larger than the largest computer that can be imagined. If you could make a model of the brain, using cells, say, the size of a volume of the *Encyclopaedia Britannica*, you would need over three-quarters of the surface of the earth to lay it out. But even if you then saw what was happening in each one of these cells – which were lighting up and which were not – you still, in your scanning of the whole vast continent of flickering lights, would not be able to tell what that brain was thinking, feeling, hoping, or dreading. You could not lead off from it wires which would, on a cathode ray tube, give you a picture of what the person was seeing or any kind of sense impression of what they were subjectively experiencing. If we want to record the brain's activity, we have to multiply it a million times to make it recordable on an electroencephalogram. Yet we do, with respect and care, pass currents of that order – that is to say a million times the brain's working current – through the brain in electrical treatment, in order to relieve it of certain patterns of thought which are painful, ridden with anguish and repetitive. For example, depression is an illness in which electrical treatment can be life-saving, and it has changed the outlook from a virtually hopeless disorder to a disorder in which 80 per cent recovery can be expected within six weeks. The fact that a great deal of the physiological approach to treatment through knowledge of neurophysiology is still empirical does not make it any the less useful. A great deal of scientific discovery was made in exactly that way and many of the advances in the neurophysiological approaches to treatment – such as giving insulin which alters the metabolism of the brain enormously and which is now largely replaced by electrical treatment and certain specific drugs which affect the conductivity within the brain – were discovered by the use of parallel types of intervention for other reasons.

Take the example of electrical treatment itself, which I think is one treatment which people need to know more about because practically everybody still talks about it as shock treatment. This is wrong: it does not produce an electric shock of a palpable kind. The patient is anaesthetised and does not experience shock of a physiological kind; nor is the patient left shocked afterwards. Indeed, the only reason it is called shock treatment is that there is a degree of physical resemblance between the apparatus used when the patient is unconscious and the kind of apparatus that people used when giving each other electric shocks as parlour games – when you used to grasp two pieces of metal, have an amp or two through your arms which gave a tingling feeling such as you might occasionally experience if you are an electrician and pick up live wires. Electrical treatment was applied as a method of treatment because of a theory which was based on a scientific observation that was wrong. The fact that many scientific observations are wrong but lead to fruitful theories has been very elegantly set up by Professor Hebb, a Fellow of the Royal Society of Canada, in a disquisition which he wrote for that Society on the contributions respectively of psychoanalysis, which is a highly refined method of pursuing the associations of random thought in human beings, and behaviourism, which is a way of observing human behaviour and drawing conclusions from it which do not necessarily depend upon communication by words at all. Hebb pointed out that although behaviourism started by being a wrong-headed theory, it has probably contributed at least as much to our understanding of learning as psychoanalysis, which was based upon a much more sophisticated concept of learning. But he also reminded his readers that all scientific hypotheses are not revealed truth, as non-scientists are apt to imagine, but are in fact sophisticated statements of ignorance, and that is what a scientific hypothesis is, and must remain, until a better one comes to replace it.

The hypothesis which originally led to electrical treatment being used was as follows. Schizophrenia is a disintegrative disorder of the personality and thought processes probably due to a disturbance in the function of the biochemistry of the brain. But schizophrenia occurs less frequently in people who also suffer from epilepsy than would be expected in view of the incidence of the two illnesses in the population as a whole. In fact the overlap was less than statistically might have been expected. So the theory was advanced that if you could give schizophrenic patients some kind of epileptic shock, or alternatively if you could give epileptics some kind of schizophrenia, you might benefit them. As it was only possible to test this hypothesis by experiment, at first animals, and then human beings, were given epileptic convulsions by having injections of a drug very much like that used to stimulate the heart. After a period of considerable discomfort, they then had an epileptic form of convulsion. We now know that this is quite unnecessary; electrical treatment does not need to produce a convulsion in order to produce beneficial results. A convulsion was a kind of indication that you had stimulated the brain sufficiently to produce the other changes. But it was found in those days that electrical treatment was far more valuable to patients who were depressed than to patients with schizophrenia. In fact electrical treatment of schizophrenia has only come back now that we have a drug which the brain can use, and which is stimulated by additional electrical reinforcement. So we now have a means of treating people based on the erroneous idea that the convulsion was good. In retrospect, with more data available, we realise that epilepsy and schizophrenia are in fact more, not less, likely to coexist than their incidence would suggest, so the whole original theory was mistaken. But the value of it is that we have a 60 to 80 per cent recovery rate within six weeks in a previously very difficult illness to treat.

Treatment by communication relies upon communicating with the patient, as in psychoanalysis or in any kind of psychotherapy, in which the patient's own method of talking is, to some extent, supplanted by free association, or a method which gives some idea of what is happening in the patient's mind below the surface. Freud's greatest contribution to medicine as a whole, and to psychiatry in particular, was to point out firstly that at least two-thirds of our instinctual behaviour, our impulses and our feelings, are inexplicable at a rational level, although we commonly give them rational explanations: and secondly that our dream world has meaning, and our waking world has part of our dream world in it; and that by studying this, we could learn more about people's total attitude to life. The psychiatrist's job is to use this kind of knowledge to bring people within the arena of communication with him, or her, and with other people. It is to bring them back. There's no magic about it. It is not a branch of medicine which has any power to produce changes in personality against the will of the patient. This is true even in the most mechanistic applications of it, for instance, neuro-surgery to prevent certain reverberating circuits within the brain from continuing. A computer also can have a reverberation circuit, whereby it will go on giving the same answer to whatever question is fed into it and it can be cleared by sending an electric impulse through it, very much as the brain can be, but when this happens you have a mechanical situation, and occasionally you may have to disconnect certain parts of the computer to put it right. When you do this in neuro-surgery, in the operation of leucotomy, what you are doing is preventing feed-back of anxiety and tension from swamping the person's response to everyday events.

Psychiatry is bound to be very heavily loaded with people's sense of values, because it deals with that most human aspect of them, their thought and their feeling. But it doesn't attempt to give them guide-lines for what those values should be. The psychiatrist is, in this sense, like any other doctor, a technician with a sense of his material, a sense of his limitations and a respect for that material. He is like somebody you call in to adjust your television set. When he has adjusted it so that you can get whatever programme you like, he does not then say, 'But you must watch BBC 2 only, because I tell you that's best for you.' Far from that, he says, 'Now the set will work, tune into whatever channel you like.' This is the psychiatrist's job. He gets your set working for you, and you decide what to do with it, so such questions as, 'Can I have a Christian psychiatrist, because I am a Christian?' or, 'Can I have a Jewish psychiatrist, because I am a Jew?' are totally irrelevant. The psychiatrist does not attempt either to guide, or to alter, your fundamental beliefs, but simply to allow you to reach them without delusions, misconceptions, and short circuits in your network, so to speak. Nevertheless, people fear that he is going to change them against their will. I put as the objective of psychiatric treatment, to restore to the individual his optimum capacity for emotional balance in maturity, for rational choice in intellectual capacity and accurate perception and interpretation of sensory experience. Those are the things you are after when you are treating somebody. Sometimes they are unattainable because the brain is wearing out, the cells are dying, the situation deteriorating. This happens to all of us if we live long enough. Then it is the psychiatrist's job to treat the relatives, to get them to show that measure of compassion and respect for what was somebody for whom they always had those feelings, because the end of somebody who is demented is pitiful and undignified, unless they are treated with that concern which once they noted and won. The psychiatrist has simply to remind people that the shell of the man or the woman is still worthy of the respect that that man or woman had ever commanded, or that men or women everywhere and always must command.

If the brain is the organ of mind, is it possible for any mechanical activity within it to account for all the creativity which is part of human beings? I mentioned the figure fifteen thousand million cells. Let us do one very rapid calculation. Take traffic lights; there are only three lights in the traffic system, they can only be on or off – red, yellow, or green. There are eight possible combinations of these lights, of which only four are used normally in traffic. But there are eight, that is, in fact, two to the power of three. From that you can deduce an elegant mathematical formula, which tells you that with any series of cells which can be either on or off, two to the power of that number will give you the total number of combinations and permutations possible. So that two to the power of fifteen thousand million, which is a staggering number, is the capacity of the brain for randomness. And it is enough for every language to be learnt by every human being, if they had the time, if they had the patience and if they knew how to use the whole of their network. We are over-endowed with capacity, but under-endowed, perhaps, with patience and determination. And the psychiatrist does not affect those things. To seek treatment is either to need it and to know that you need it, or to be brought for it because you cannot find your way around to it. But it is not, in any way, to be more contemptible, or more foolish, than someone who has leukaemia or someone who has cancer of the lung.

In conclusion, the psychiatrist's job is not only to restore either the respect of the patient, or his own system and network, but to give him the freedom of choice of how much of this capacity he will use. People are afraid of things like brain-washing. Brain-washing is merely a vulgar term for an extremely hideous thing; that is, the ability to damage the function of the brain, so that temporarily it functions as though it were disturbed out of its normal network of communication. But the rigidity, the limitation, the inflexibility of the brain-washed person are those of someone who is mentally ill and are so detectable, and except in the witness box, or in the court where they say their set piece, they are obviously ill, and this illness can be cured and does get better. To say that you can make people ill by mistreating them is only to say what we all know, and the psychiatrist's task is always to make people better, not to make them ill, and not to influence them, but to set them free.

WINCH I take it that my role here should be to ask questions. Perhaps the greatest difficulty in this subject is to find precisely the right questions to ask, rather than the difficulty of finding answers. I don't mean by that that when the questions have been asked, the answers will necessarily be easy to come by: what I do mean is that the biggest difficulty lies in seeing exactly what is problematic about a sphere like that of psychiatric treatment.

My first question then is this: Why should the subject of psychiatric treatment be made a topic on its own in a series of this sort about morals and medicine? After all, one wouldn't expect to find physiotherapy, or gynaecology down on the programme. I know that there has been a discussion of abortion – but that's a different matter, for there are, of course, special problems there. There are not, however, problems arising simply out of the fact that gynaecology is regarded as a branch of medicine. I do think, though, that the feeling that probably lay behind including psychiatric treatment as a subject for discussion has some justification. It is the feeling that we cannot regard psychiatry as just a species of the genus medicine, as perhaps we might regard gynaecology as a species of that genus. For, in bringing the conditions with which psychiatrists deal under the heading of medicine, in regarding these problems as medical problems at all, already difficulties are involved, difficulties which raise ethical issues.

My first point is, then, that to regard the kind of difficulty that psychiatric patients are in as a species of difficulty that can be treated medically, is already to make a move, the nature of which is problematic. I am choosing my words carefully at this point. I am not asserting dogmatically that the move in question is a mistaken one. It is a move that has been made and one which has had widely ramified consequences in the way we think about all sorts of human problems. I mean only that, in coming to think of mental troubles as a suitable subject for medical treatment, a conceptual move has been made, the nature of which is not immediately clear. If I could take an analogy from another sphere to illustrate my point: in mathematics, difficulties of a conceptual nature arise when you start asking questions about infinity, and the question could be asked: can infinity be treated like a number? And, of course, if you do try to treat it like other sorts of number, you get into serious difficulties. Or, again, if you think of irrational numbers or imaginary numbers in mathematics, these share some of the properties of more familiar examples of the notion of number; others they don't share, however, and if one is not careful in how one treats these things, one gets into tangles. My point about psychiatry is that one has to be careful about this in the same sort of way. Certainly there are very many respects in which the problems of patients dealt with by psychiatrists are unavoidably seen as falling into the province of medicine. Nevertheless, there are features of those problems which, I suggest, cause difficulty if thought of in this way. But, of course, it is a fact that we do now think of these problems from that point of view, and I am not suggesting that we should go back on that; I don't even think it would make sense to suggest that we should. This is something which is part of our culture now, and my point is only that we should try to be clear about where it has brought us.

Yet there are obstacles in the way of even trying to get clear about this. The very idea of mental disorder is threatening to us: the fear that one could suffer it, that one's very personality could be subject to dissolution from within, is in many ways an even more disturbing thought than that it is subject to dissolution in death. I emphasise the 'from within'. So it is very tempting to hold it at arm's length, out of harm's way as it were. And I suggest that talk about health and illness and medical treatment in this context may, in certain circumstances, be a method of doing this. In saying that, I don't want to contradict anything that Dr Stafford-Clark has said, in many of his published writings, about the increase in humaneness in the treatment of psychic disorders, which has gone along with regarding them as falling squarely within the medical domain. What he says about that seems to me quite right. The more humaneness there is in this sphere, as in any other sphere, the better. I want to say only that there's another side to this picture, too, and that other ways of thinking about psychic disorder may make it possible to see certain things that the representation of it in purely medical terms obscures.

Talk about health and sickness has often been used in a metaphorical way. For example, in Plato's treatment of ethical questions you will find considerable play made with the idea of evil-doing as involving a sickness of the soul; and with the notion of punishment as involving a treatment and possibly a cure of that sickness. I mention that here because it's very clear that Plato was speaking metaphorically (I don't, as a matter of fact, think it was a very useful metaphor in the context, but that would be another subject). Whereas, of course, when these days we talk about mental sickness, in the sense in which psychiatrists deal with mental sickness, we don't take ourselves to be using a metaphor. Now Plato was not advocating that evil-doers should be handed over to doctors. That wasn't the point of the medical analogy there at all. So when we talk about psychiatric disorders as falling within the medical sphere we are not using a metaphor as Plato was.

The difficulty in the way of seeing exactly what we are doing is exacerbated by the very wide diversity to be found within the sphere of what we call mental ailments. We have cases in which straightforwardly physical symptoms like paralysis of limbs, or deafness, or blindness, are found not to stem from straightforward physical causes, but from what we call 'mental' causes. I am thinking here particularly of Freud's first steps towards the development of psychoanalytic theory, when he found that certain physical paralyses were not explicable in an ordinary neurological way, but required reference to the patient's understanding of the function of the paralysed limb. Again, we have cases of the sort that Dr Stafford-Clark has mentioned, where symptoms of an unambiguously mental sort, like melancholia or paranoia, are treated by physical means, by means of electro-convulsive treatment, pills, injections of various sorts and so on. We have cases of functional disorder of the perceptual system, hallucinations and what-not. Finally, we have cases of what I shall call, no doubt very unprofessionally, disordered thinking.

It is the last type of case which gives rise to the most serious problems from my point of view. One has to ask here what sense one can attach to the notion of 'disorder', as applied to thinking, and at what point disorder in thinking becomes a clinical and medical matter. To go into this question thoroughly, it would be necessary to spend quite a bit of time trying to say in general how one distinguishes between health and sickness – and I don't mean just in the mental sphere, I mean in the physical sphere, too. It is not by any means easy to say what one means by health and sickness, even when simply talking about the body. But let us consider some problems that arise when we try to make that distinction in the mental sphere.

Obviously the concept of the normal, and the distinction between what is normal and what is abnormal, is important here. But what does that mean? One way in which normality is distinguished from abnormality, for instance, in relation to organs of the human body, has to do with the function of such organs. If you were talking about a normal hand, as distinct from an abnormal hand, you would have at some point to make reference to the role that the hand plays in the working of the total human organism – the function it fulfils in the organism's activities. That does not settle the matter, though, because were you to ask what kind of activities, you would presumably have to say, 'its normal activities', and the problem is back at the beginning.

The mind, however, is not an organ. Dr Stafford-Clark suggested that we might perhaps regard the brain as the organ of the mind. I would not want to talk about it in that way. But he, rightly, was not inclined to talk about the mind itself as an organ. The mind in that respect is not like the brain, although of course disorders in the brain may give rise to mental disorders. Talking about a person's mind is one way of talking about *him,* in a sense in which talking about a person's hands is not in the same way talking about him. There is no function which everybody could agree is the function of man. Men are not defined by a function, as are human organs; though in connection with perceptual disorders, such as hallucinations, I suppose the notion of function would come in and it would come in also in connection with hysterical paralysis and the like. But I am thinking rather of difficulties arising in applying the categories of health and sickness to instances of what is sometimes called deviant behaviour.

The ethical importance of this point is that any explicit definition of man's function would be in an important sense ethically arbitrary and would involve taking sides in controversial ethical issues. A point Dr Stafford-Clark made is relevant here. He emphasised, quite rightly, that it is not part of the function of a psychiatrist to say what a patient's values should be. In this respect he is a sort of technician. Dr Stafford-Clark compared him to a television technician who says: 'Now the set will work, do what you like with it.' So the patient decides how he is to live after he has regained his health. I want to suggest that questions about values come in at another point. They do not simply arise in the context of treatment. They also come in in the context of deciding who is to be regarded as in need of treatment in the first place. Here I should like to read the description of a case mentioned by a psychiatrist in Dublin, Dr Drury – this is one of his own patients:

> This case came to my notice over fifteen years ago when many of the methods of treatment we now have were not known. Mr D. was 67 years of age. A retired civil servant. A man of great piety who devoted his retirement to prayer and works of charity. His wife had no sympathy for what she regarded as a morbid religiousness. One morning at Mass, he heard read the words of the Gospel, 'Go and sell all that thou hast and give to the poor, and thou shalt have treasure in Heaven, and come and follow Me'. These words spoke to Mr D, like a command. And straightaway he left the church, putting all the money that was on him into the poor-box at the door. He set off to walk the 135 miles to Lough Derg, a famous place of pilgrimage in Ireland since earliest times. When he did not return for his breakfast and the morning passed without news of him his wife became alarmed and notified the Guards. Eventually, that evening, he was stopped by a policeman of a small village about thirty miles from Dublin. He was seen by a doctor and put on a temporary certificate for admission to a mental hospital. He made no protest at entering hospital, told his story clearly, and accepted what had happened as God's will. I informed the Medical Superintendent the next morning that we had admitted a saint.

I imagine that many psychiatrists faced with this case might have taken quite a different view of the matter. The question of whether or not a person in a condition of this sort should be treated medically, is itself one, I suggest, that involves ethical decisions. This is a different point from the question of interfering with, or imposing values on, a patient once he has accepted treatment, once he is under treatment. It may be said that this difficulty is overcome as long as the people who come for treatment do so voluntarily – except for those who, as Dr Stafford-Clark put it, just cannot find their way in life at all. But I don't think this entirely removes one's disquiet at what is involved in this issue.

We must not forget that the line people will take when faced with fundamental difficulties in their lives, whether they will regard these as calling for treatment of a medical sort or not – depends a great deal on the climate of thought in which they move. In so far as there is a climate in which it is thought, as a matter of course, that fundamental difficulties of a certain sort about one's life, do fall within the psychiatric sphere, then people are more likely to seek that kind of help than otherwise, and it may well be that in doing so they will return to 'normal and happy lives' sooner than they otherwise would. It is certainly entirely possible, even likely, that their difficulties will be got rid of more efficiently that way than they would if they were left to find their own way through them. But to lose a problem is not to solve it, and in many cases there are situations in which a man just cannot find his way about in life at all. Dr Drury, in the paper I quoted from, also cites the case of Tolstoy who, at one time of his life, exhibited symptoms which certainly had a psychiatric look about them, though he found his way through them without benefit of medical assistance and developed as a writer in the way he did as an outcome of those problems.

The question I want to raise is, When is one justified in such cases in deciding that a person is in a situation calling for medical treatment, and what sort of decision is that?

The Chairman, Lord Cohen, then invited the two speakers to put questions to each other and opened the discussion to the audience.

STAFFORD-CLARK First of all I would like to dispose of two matters on which Professor Winch is a little uneasy, which I think can be cleared up. They have to do with the use of Greek words. The Greeks talked about the *psyche,* meaning by this the intelligence and possibly the personality. They talked about the *pneuma*, meaning the soul or the spirit. A psychiatrist, straight from the Greek, is a doctor, an *iatros*, a physician who is concerned with the *psyche*, which is the intelligence and the personality and with the way in which the person who possesses those uses them. So that a psychiatrist is not concerned with problems of the soul. I have great sympathy with Dr Drury who, on encountering a gentleman who wished to give all his goods to the poor and with no other sign of thought disorder, was doubtful whether that man was a case for diagnosis at all. The diagnosis of thought disorder is a diagnosis which doctors make with certain rules which work tolerably well and I will try if you like to instance them to you and ask Professor Winch whether they make his task any easier.

Thought disorder is not simply thinking differently from other people. Thought disorder, as far as the psychiatrist is concerned, is either an interruption of the stream of thought (such as thought block, with which most of us are familiar when we are tired); or you lose your train of thought and think along lines which do not seem any longer to be governed by yourself; or you have ideas of being influenced in your thinking, getting sensory information which is not perceived by anybody else and which you discover, to your dismay very often, is peculiar to you – hearing voices, having thoughts enter your mind which you cannot control and which seem to you to be coming from outside. Or you may have concrete thinking.

A good example of concrete thinking is when you ask someone about proverbs: you ask them if they know any proverbs and they often say 'Yes'. Then you say, 'Well, do you for example know the proverb, "people who live in glass houses shouldn't throw stones"?' And they say 'Yes'. Then you say, 'Well, what does it mean?' If they have the form of thought disorder known as concrete thinking, they might reply, 'Well, if you throw stones you break the glass.' Then you say, 'Does it have a more general meaning?' And they say, 'Yes, you shouldn't throw rocks from outside either, because that breaks the glass too.' They are being perfectly logical, but they are limited by an inability for abstract conceptual thought with which to enlighten the problem. So, for example, you might say: ' "A stitch in time saves nine" – do you know that one?' 'Yes, I do.' 'What does it mean?' 'Well, it means that if you don't stitch up a rent in your pocket it gets bigger.' 'Does it have any more general meaning?' Then they may say either, 'Well, it could apply to your socks', or they may just say, 'I don't understand what you mean.' Now that is thought disorder as a doctor encounters it.

The inability to remember, the inability to repeat a sentence from memory or to hold digits in one's mind to the point of being unable even to remember, for example, what one has read in a book from page to page – these are the sort of things that psychiatrists deal with. They do not deal with vagaries of behaviour unless these vagaries leave the person sufficiently lost and bewildered as to be, from the psychiatrist's point of view, disabled. I don't know whether I have reassured Professor Winch at all, but I do not think there is an ethical problem about regarding psychiatry as a part of medicine.

One other problem on which perhaps Professor Winch might like either to enlighten me, or to ask for enlightenment if I can give it, is that of responsibility. There is an uneasy feeling that if the mechanics of the brain are directly related to the actual process of thinking, then the brain is an organ which must work in some mechanical way, which makes the randomness I described earlier hard to conceive. People then go on to say: 'If the brain works in a mechanical way, surely we can't know that it works at all.' Professor J. B. S. Haldane put this idea very elegantly when he said, 'If all my thoughts are due to the behaviour of electrical charges within my brain, like the behaviour of billiard balls on a table are due to the direction in which they are struck, then how can I have any thoughts which are valid about my brain; how do I know that truth exists; how, in fact, am I aware of anything?' But most people take it for granted that their consciousness, judgement, memory and interpretation are working, until they feel them go wrong, in the same way as they might feel they have got toothache. That's the point at which they go to their doctor who, if he is enlightened, perhaps refers them to a psychiatrist and if he isn't, tells them not to worry!

WINCH On Dr Stafford-Clark's first point: there are indeed many cases of thought disorder where no one would have any hesitation in saying that here was sickness, here was something that needed treatment, and Dr Stafford-Clark has given examples of the kind of symptoms that psychiatrists look for along those lines. However, surely he would not deny that there are difficult borderline cases where the question, 'Is it a case for treatment?' seriously presents itself and has no easy answer. Of course talk about 'disorder' here raises difficult problems. At the end of the list of various kinds of disorder; interruption of one's stream of thought, thinking along lines not governed by oneself, the idea that one's being controlled by some alien force, difficulties in judgement and so on, at the end of this you used the phrase 'someone who is sufficiently lost and bewildered to come to the psychiatrist for help'. But one may be lost and bewildered in relation to many situations in life. One may not be able to see one's way about at all; one may be in a situation where one's no longer able to understand even what one's problems are. If one is in such a situation, does that sound like a description of a case of someone who needs psychiatric treatment?

STAFFORD-CLARK The process of assessing whether a patient needs treatment is one in which the patient and the doctor mutually participate. The first thing that a good doctor has to do is to listen to the patient. It has always been the role of the doctor, as well as the lawyer, the accountant, the bank manager, and the priest, to listen to people in trouble. Occasionally I have heard colleagues of mine say, and I have said myself: 'Dear sir or madam, what you need, I think, in this situation is a good lawyer and not me.' Because the trouble is one of conjugal disagreement in which property rights and so forth are being bandied about and the psychiatrist may feel that whereas people are being, to use a popular phrase, bloody-minded to each other, there is nothing the matter with their capacity to alter their behaviour if they so wish. So I think doctors can also allow patients to show them whether they suffer from thought disorder or not. A colleague of mine once wrote in an essay, in a symposium on psychiatry and religion, that if, for example, you take a single experience which would seem to be delusional, or hallucinatory to everybody else – for instance Joan of Arc hearing voices – then that doesn't have to be diagnosed as an illness if in every other way she shows no evidence of other thought disorder or of an altered relationship to the rest of the world and a disturbance of her personality.

A doctor can decide, though he may not always be right, if he can help. He can decide whether his help is needed within three-quarters of an hour of letting a patient talk to him; at the end of that time he will have been able to make a diagnosis. And I still don't know whether, in the case of Mr D., Dr Drury or the policeman or medical superintendent, were right. It is quite possible that Mr D. knew exactly what he was doing and decided that he was going to take the Bible literally and that was his decision. It doesn't make him a mental case thereby.

Members of the audience then posed questions to the speakers.

JOHN D. FLETCHER I would like to follow up this question of distinguishing between the normal and the abnormal in all sorts of respects, but I should particularly like to ask where does persuasion end and brain-washing begin? And, further, is either or both in any instance morally justifiable and where do religious conversions stand with respect to either of these?

STAFFORD-CLARK Obviously I can't give you a full answer to that in a limited space of time, but I can give you a reference or two. If you read William Sargant's book *Battle for the Mind*[1] you will get one answer to the question of what brain-washing is. This is based on the theory that brain-washing is to human beings what conditioning is either to human beings or to animals: the evocation of various responses by various types of stimuli so that an original response is evoked by a new kind of stimulus. Pavlov showed that dogs whose mouths watered naturally when they were confronted with meat could be induced to have their mouths water by ringing a bell, if you showed the meat and rang the bell at the same time, say two or three times a day, and after that just rang the bell. If, after a time, you then kept on varying the stimuli, it was lost in the dog's capacity to respond appropriately. The dog might then show a paradoxical response of perhaps snarling, or struggling when the bell was rung, or the light flashed, or whatever the conditioning response was, if the expected food didn't arrive. Sargant really suggested, in his book, that the brain is a system purely of reflexes which can be reversed by paradoxical inhibition and stimulation. The arguments against this are put forward in reviews of the book, including my own. I concluded that whereas it is perfectly possible, without physically torturing people, to break up their rhythm, their sleep, their normal response and stimuli, and encourage them in the view that if they will express a totally different opinion to that which they already hold, they will not only be better, but will be saved, then you can convert them temporarily. But this is inducing a form of mental illness. In fact it is a refined form of torture. As such it is obviously unethical in my view. Simple persuasion, however, is to attempt, by communicating with someone, to get them to see your point of view and possibly to alter their own in the light of it. This is no part of a psychiatrist's job, but it is part of a human being's relationship with other human beings. If it were not possible to persuade people, no one would ever be, for example, either seduced on the one hand, or converted on the other. The ethics of conversion and seduction are different, but they are both products of a kind of persuasion that either works or doesn't.

[1] William Sargant, *Battle for the Mind* (Heinemann, 1957).

H. E. TITCHMARSH Would Dr Stafford-Clark please say what part hypnosis has in psychiatric treatment?

STAFFORD-CLARK It constitutes, I would say, a valuable fifteen per cent of all treatment, not more. It is a technique for gaining a rather less critical acceptance of information from the person who is imposing it than would otherwise be the case. Its value in medicine is that people's response to their environment, and to themselves, can be altered to relieve stress. For example, states of anxiety that have become associated with certain situations, what are known technically as phobias, can be altered if the person can be taught first of all to relax sufficiently, muscularly, to a critical point at which his state of mobilisation drops below that at which he is aware of fear, so instead he becomes calm. This can be produced in a consulting room by hypnosis, in which simple suggestions of calmness and relaxation and confidence are made, and then these, once acquired, can be reinforced with the patient's willing co-operation to a point where the patient can become calm very rapidly and very easily. Very often you can condition this response, if the patient is willing, by giving him a code word to which, having learned how to gain this calmness, he will instantly respond, without losing consciousness or in any way becoming unable to manage his day-to-day conduct of affairs. Hypnosis can also be used to produce a lowered sensibility to pain, in a dentist's chair, for example, and during childbirth, as in Grantley Dick Reid's methods of relaxation during childbirth.

I think that it has been satisfactorily proved that you can hypnotise people against their will only if they are sufficiently afraid of the idea that they are already highly suggestible. If they are not in the least interested, you cannot hypnotise them unless they wish to be hypnotised, and indeed a lot of people cannot be hypnotised anyway, because they will not give that amount of concentration to the evocation of calmness, or quietness, or inner peace, or whatever it is that you are using as your starting point. They won't even relax. Lots of people can relax and can be taught to relax, but unless they will, you can't hypnotise them. Another question is, can you, if you do hypnotise them with their consent, make them do things which they would not otherwise do? The answer is only to the extent that they will accept your responsibility rather than their own, which is back to the question of persuasion. For example, if you say to them, 'You will now go out in the street and shoot the first person you meet,' hypnosis will not induce them to do that, but if you say, 'You will slap your wife's face. You've never done it before, it's time you did,' you may just tip the balance then. This is only part of the art of medicine and it has no magic about it. That's the really important thing. People are afraid of hypnosis because they believe it is a kind of magic, but in fact it is the other way round. A lot of magic in primitive communities is a kind of hypnosis.

N. S. BARNETT I feel that a question raised by Professor Winch might well be answered by Dr Stafford-Clark, and that is, 'Would the light of Tolstoy still have shone upon the world if there had been psychiatrists in the offing?'

STAFFORD-CLARK I'm sure it would. You see, psychiatrists, like all other human beings, are not without their faults, but they do not seek to take over and treat people who are doing all right anyway. Eccentricity has never been a cause for psychiatric treatment.

WINCH But the point about Tolstoy was that at a certain time he wasn't doing all right by any means: he was in a pretty bad way.

STAFFORD-CLARK If Tolstoy had been depressed and unable to write and had then been treated, he would resume writing afterwards and be better. I can think of, for instance, a quite brilliant cartoonist who could not draw or have any ideas for drawings when he was depressed, but who, after appropriate psychological and physiological treatment, regained his form. I can think of the same thing applying to judges and teachers that I have known as patients of colleagues, or occasionally patients of mine, but when they have come for treatment, they have come because their doctor has felt that they were disabled from their normal capacity, and Tolstoy's light shone when he was well. When he was feeling anguish and revulsion at the world's predicament, he could still sometimes communicate this and sometimes not. When he couldn't, I think psychiatry might have helped him to communicate. When he could, he had no need of it.

T. KELLY Robert Louis Stephenson, in one of his essays, compared the electrician who was a new phenomenon in his day, much as a psychiatrist is in ours, with the Creator. '*Fiat lux*,' says the sedate electrician, and there is light. I have admired Dr Stafford-Clark's confident exposition enormously, but I should like to ask him, on behalf of a lot of lay people, whether he does not sometimes feel qualms about his God-like ability to manipulate people and, in some degree, to change their personalities.

STAFFORD-CLARK Well, my answer to that is instant and total disavowal of that ability. I cannot change anyone's personality. All I can do is to enable that personality to function perhaps a little bit more in the way that they and those who know them would recognise as being characteristic of them at their best. That's all I can do, and I would say, on behalf of psychiatrists as a whole, that such confidence that we display is the whistling in the dark which doctors are normally expected to do for the sake of people who are frightened of being ill in the presence of someone who is supposed to be able to help.

G. ABRAHAMS Dr Stafford-Clark spoke of himself as a person who repaired mental machinery and I understood from his description that this was a cognitive machinery. But it occurs to me that Dr Stafford-Clark must have to do much with those who are volitionally feeble; persons who have a taste for stealing and call themselves kleptomaniacs, or persons with a taste for homicide, and in that connection, I would ask one question: Does Dr Stafford-Clark find the concept of wickedness to be a useful one in his subject?

STAFFORD-CLARK I don't think any psychiatrist, as a psychiatrist, is able to dismiss the reality of evil in the world. I was asked once by Lord Packenham, when he was conducting a research on behalf of the Nuffield Foundation into the causes of crime, whether I thought there was such a thing as medical crime and I said that I thought that perhaps fifteen per cent of the acts which were criminal were committed by people whose physical and mental health was sufficiently impaired to induce them to commit these acts, but that the other eighty-five per cent were committed by healthy people. The majority of people who commit acts of violence are temporarily very upset and disturbed, but they are not ill, necessarily; because you can't stand somebody and so you do them a violent injury, this does not automatically make you a sick person. It may merely mean that the amount of control which you have exercised is less than the best of which you are capable, and highly regrettable. There is no conflict between the empirical concept of free will and the psychiatrist's function to improve emotional, cognitive and behavioural states within the limits of that person's personality.

WINCH Some time ago Dr Stafford-Clark organised and took part in a series of television programmes called, 'Mind and Motive', in which use was made of juxtapositions of clinical cases from psychiatric practice against, for instance, cases of mob behaviour in connection with racialism and so on. The suggestion seemed to be that there was some connection here between such social manifestations and what can be learnt in the psychiatrist's consulting room. Dr Stafford-Clark was making, and I should like to ask him now if there was any claim here, and if so, what it was.

STAFFORD-CLARK I think the claim is one that is learned from the degree of disturbance of judgement which one sees in people who are ill. For example, some mechanisms, which exist in most of us, resist the idea of change or difference in our society; some people believe quite firmly that anyone who is not of them is against them. If they are mentally ill, they will believe that the whole world is against them, or that there are organised conspiracies on a world scale against them, or that the people in the houses all up and down the street are against them. This kind of illness has, as its rationalisation, very much the same kind of support as the view that, for example, to have people from another part of the world coming and living here is intrinsically a bad thing. What we were trying to do in that television series, was to show that self-preservation motives can lead people to behave both cruelly and unjustly when they are psychotic and when they are normal, but that the rationalisations which they use to defend this will be quite similar in both cases.

J. SAVITZ Is psychological pain a reality? It was a common phenomenon some time ago to describe inexplicable symptoms of pain and discomfort as being psychological.

STAFFORD-CLARK The answer is that pain is real if you feel it. The only reality which we can grant to pain is that it is felt. If you have a pain in your head, or your foot, or your tooth, and you come and tell me, and I tell you you haven't got that pain, because after X-raying it I can see no abnormality, then it is I who am a fool, and you who are misjudged. What I try and teach medical students are two things. There are two kinds of pain, which do not correspond to local structural lesions. One, is what we call central pain, where the brain is acting obviously abnormally; and this is the kind of pain you get in the phantom limb of the amputee. They feel pain in their arm after it has been amputated. The area of the brain which deals with that part of the limb is still, as it were, in a turmoil and that turmoil is interpreted and felt as pain. And there is another kind of pain, which you can have simply because your brain generally is under stress and you are suffering, and you may experience this as pain. But the only criterion of whether pain is real or not is whether you really feel it or not. The only unreal pain is the pain that you claim to feel, when you know you don't feel it, for reasons which may be devious, or difficult to discover, but are imaginable.

COHEN There are one or two points, which perhaps I might reasonably make by way of summary. They are really answers to certain questions which have been posed. The first is, 'How do we distinguish between health and sickness?' The answer, of course, is that these are purely man-made conceptions. It is man who classifies phenomena, not God. We have said that there is a certain range of bodily structure, of bodily function, of bodily feeling which may be regarded as normal. Beyond that everyone might recognise that which is abnormal, although, of course, there is the in-between bit, which may, or may not be – and this depends upon what limits you put to normality. We are all sometimes a little depressed, or sometimes elated, but I doubt if we feel those emotions beyond what might be called the normal range. The same is true of organic disease. What is the normal blood pressure? When is a high blood pressure to be regarded as manifestation of disease? When can it be regarded as within normal limits? These are all questions which refer, as I say, to the organic as well as the psychical. It is also true to say that no disease is wholly physical, and no disease is wholly psychological. This again is because psychological and physical are man-made terms. They happen to be convenient classifications for certain purposes.

Of course, we have not reached the end of the road in our understanding of problems of psychiatry and sometimes there are associated ethical problems. But certainly some of the anxieties which have been expressed about psychiatric treatment will have been dispelled by the very clear words used by Dr Stafford-Clark, and Professor Winch, on the problems which confront those undertaking psychiatric treatment.

VI GENETICS AND MORAL RESPONSIBILITY

C. O. CARTER & BERNARD WILLIAMS

CARTER I am going to deal with two quite different aspects of genetics and moral responsibility. The first aspect is, I think, the more important one; this is the moral responsibility that we in this generation have for the genetic health of the next generation and the generation after that. The second aspect is perhaps less important, but may be of more interest as a topic for discussion and disagreement; this is the extent to which the control of an individual's development, by the interaction of his genetic endowment and his environmental experiences, predetermines his behaviour and so limits the extent to which he has moral responsibility for this behaviour. Taking first our responsibility for the genetic endowment of the next generation: Almost everyone, in a culture such as our own, accepts that we do have a responsibility to provide, so far as we can, a good environment for our children. This we are all agreed on. The main responsibility here lies with individual parents, but it is also accepted that the community as a whole has a responsibility to provide those forms of training which are best given communally. For example, education in schools. It is also accepted that in many instances where the parents are failing badly in their bringing-up of the children, and in particular, where there's actual danger to the child's life, that the child must be taken away into community care. This is, I think, straightforward. As regards genetic endowment, I believe that our increasing knowledge in human genetics does bring a responsibility to use this knowledge too in the interests of the coming generations. Once again the real responsibility here lies with the individual parental couples, who should, I think, in planning how many children they will have, or indeed sometimes whether they have children at all, give due consideration to the kind of genetic factors, or genes, they are likely to pass on to their children. I say likely to pass on, because there is a built-in uncertainty in hereditary transmission. This depends on

Mendel's first law, that our hereditary factors or genes are in pairs, and a parent only passes on one member of each pair to a particular child. The choice of which member of a pair is transmitted to a particular child is a purely random one, like the outcome, heads or tails, of tossing a coin. Mendel's second law states that the selection from one pair of genes is largely independent of the selection from any other pair. So it is really like tossing up hundreds of coins at once. A parent will pass on half his hereditary factors to a child; he cannot obviously pass on a gene he has not himself got, but he can transmit a great variety of different combinations from the thousands of gene-pairs he, or she, possesses. So hereditary transmission is essentially a matter of probabilities, and these probabilities must guide parents, I maintain, in deciding the size of their families. Such decisions on family size have, of course, now been made possible, but only recently been made possible, by the development of highly effective methods of family planning, appropriate to different religious persuasions, such that it is now virtually possible to plan the birth of each child. Whether the community as a whole, in addition to individual parents, has any direct responsibility for the genetic endowment of children, I very much doubt. The community does have a responsibility to make the means of family planning available to all parents, so that they can plan the size of their families, and there is still quite a bit to be done here. The community also has a responsibility to make information available to parents through medical genetic clinics and other means, in such a way that parents do have the knowledge on which to base sensible decisions on family size. Direct community action, however, in this field has very real dangers, not only from the point of view of ethics, but also from the danger of unwise, or too narrow a choice of genetic objectives. The responsibility does, and should, lie with the parents and I do doubt if there is any exception to this principle.

Now, this parental responsibility has several different aspects. One consideration in planning family size must, of course, be the actual rate of population growth. I don't think, as far as Britain is concerned, that there is yet any real cause for anxiety here. We are not in danger of a population explosion in this country, and the indications are that when all children are planned, the birth rate will be very little, if at all, in excess of replacement rate. These population aspects, however, have little directly to do with genetics, except that if the number of children born in each generation is, as must ultimately be, very close to replacement rate, then it does make it all the more desirable that as few as possible of such children as are born should carry genetic predisposition to physical, or mental handicaps. If average family size should be only a little over two children per parental couple, the genetic responsibilities of parents are such that this average should be made up of a considerable variety of family sizes, with some parents planning considerably larger families than two, and some parents planning only one child, or occasionally deciding to have no child of their own at all.

The genetic considerations that should increasingly influence parents in planning a family size may be divided into medical and social, though the distinction is not a rigid one, and the two categories overlap. The medical considerations have been highlighted by the remarkable success of the environmental health services in reducing environmental causes of childhood death, morbidity, and handicap. The major part of such morbidity, illness, and handicap is now in whole, or considerable part, genetically determined. This is a new development over the last twenty years. For example, about half of all cases of congenital blindness, and about a half of all cases of congenital deafness, are genetically determined by mutant genes, mostly recessive. About a third of all instances of severe mental retardation are due to a single chromosome anomaly, the extra G chromosome responsible for Mongolism, and about a tenth are due to mutant genes of large effect, causing inborn biochemical errors. Further, the two most serious and common groups of congenital malformations, those of brain, and spinal cord, especially spina bifida, and anencephaly, and the congenital malformations of the heart, have a complex multi-factorial causation, but there are clear indications that this causation includes a substantial, if complex, genetic component.

All these conditions, except for Mongolism, are to some extent treatable, but prevention of the birth of such children is obviously most desirable. Such prevention will come in various ways. One way is going to be the detection of parents at special risk of having such children, and warning them of the risk; for example, the one-in-four risk of a recessive condition, when both parents carry the mutant gene concerned. The advice here is a medical responsibility, but the decision, the responsibility of whether to take, say, a one-in-four risk of a congenitally deaf, or blind child, or whether to adopt a child instead, rests with the parents. We know from experience that parents on the whole take sensible decisions on this. Another method – a method of control rather than prevention, which will become of major importance for conditions due to chromosome abnormalities, and in some instances to conditions due to mutant genes – is going to be the detection of the abnormality early in a pregnancy, followed by the offer to the parents of an abortion if they want it. The techniques are, as yet, experimental and not generally available, but early results are already encouraging, and I think it is going to be possible within twenty years to offer such a screening to all parents early in the pregnancy as a routine procedure. The choice before parents will be whether they should ask for such tests – they won't be forced on them – and then whether they should ask for a termination of the pregnancy if it is certain, or at least highly probable that the results of the pregnancy will be, for example, a child with severe mental retardation. The potential effect of such a procedure, if proved safe and once the facilities are available, is great. The birth of children with Mongolism would be very largely prevented, since very few parents would not wish to avail themselves of an offer of termination in this particular condition. The decision on termination would be more difficult for the parents, where, for example, the foetus was found to be a male with an extra Y chromosome, which as I will mention later, gives a yet unknown, but certainly substantially increased risk, not of physical abnormality, but of severe behaviour disorder: or where the foetus was found to be a male with an extra X chromosome, and so will be sterile, have an increased risk of behaviour disorder, and also an increased risk of mild mental retardation as well. These are obviously going to be quite difficult ethical problems. So much then for some of the medical aspects.

Turning now to the genetics of socially valuable qualities. A quality such as intelligence, as measured by intelligence tests, is certainly potentially socially valuable. Our debt to those with good brains who use them in the community interest is enormous. In contrast it is difficult, and is going to become increasingly difficult as our society becomes more complex, for individuals who have difficulty in acquiring any sort of skill to fit happily into society. The need now in industry is not only to be skilled but to be able to acquire several new skills during the course of one's working life. A substantial proportion of the variation in intelligence in a population is due to genetic variation: there is no doubt about this, although you cannot estimate the proportion very precisely within a population and also the proportion will vary from one population to another. The proportion of the variation that is genetic in Britain is almost certainly higher than in the culturally more heterogeneous society of the United States where there are considerably bigger environmental differences than we have here. There are strong indications that several, perhaps many, pairs of genes are involved in the genetic control of the development of intelligence and for this reason and also, no doubt, in part because of common family environment, children in a family tend to develop intelligence levels related to the mid-parental average. But, because of the segregation of the genes I mentioned earlier, children may deviate considerably up or down from this average. Because of gene segregation, too, highly intelligent children can come from parents of quite average intelligence. However, intelligent children are found in highest proportion, though not necessarily in highest absolute numbers, among the offspring of intelligent parents. Conversely children who are mentally retarded, but not severely so, are found in highest proportion among the offspring of parents who are themselves of below average intelligence. Other things being equal it is in our social interest then that intelligent parents should aim at an average family size of more than two children and dull parents, parents below average intelligence, aim at two children or less. Once again it is the responsibility of the parents and not a field for Government action. Most encouragingly, there are strong indications in many countries including Britain, United States, France, and Germany that with respect to planned children the more intelligent the parents, the more children they have. Given the opportunity for planning, parents are taking sensible decisions on family size in relation to the likely intelligence levels in their children, just as they do on the medical probabilities.

To turn more briefly to my other theme: genetics and determinism. The biologist is used to thinking of a child's development as depending on a continuing interaction of his genetic endowment with the environment the child experiences. This viewpoint is deterministic, and raises the question of the extent to which an individual has any real choice in developing his personality and controlling his behaviour. We do, of course, accept that a psychotic individual – in layman's language a madman – such as a schizophrenic or manic depressive is usually not responsible for his behaviour. It is also accepted that an individual who is severely mentally retarded is not responsible for his behaviour. But both environmental and genetic factors may also predispose to abnormal and socially 'dangerous' behaviour patterns not associated with psychosis or severe mental retardation. A genetically determined example is the behaviour disturbances associated with the extra Y chromosome to which I referred above. This is a truly genetic condition present at conception: though it is due to a fresh mutation and is not inherited from either parent. It is genetic but not inherited. We do not know yet what proportion of XYY individuals develop behaviour disorders – some are leading normal lives. But certainly the risk of developing a psychopathic personality is much higher for them than for males of the ordinary XY chromosome pattern. A very rough estimate would be that at present an XYY individual has something like thirty times the probability of a normal male, of ending up in a maximum security institution.

Examples of behaviour disorders that are in the main environmentally determined are those one sees following damage to the brain, particularly that associated with temporal lobe epilepsy. Here, too, these delinquent individuals appear in otherwise quite normal families. In other instances of delinquent behaviour cultural factors are clearly most important. The individual and his family may belong to a criminal sub-culture and though there is no genetic abnormality, and there is no environmentally caused brain damage, one suspects that here too the abnormal behaviour is equally predetermined. This deterministic viewpoint cannot, I think, be proved. It is open to anyone to believe in a soul which has some power of choice and decision beyond the limitations imposed by heredity and environment. But if we do accept the deterministic viewpoint, that genes and environment determine whether an individual faced with a choice of behaviour does or does not think about its likely consequences and particularly the likely effect on others, what are some of the consequences? Punishment for criminal behaviour then must, I think, be regarded as cruelty unless it has therapeutic value in inducing more desirable behaviour patterns. Detention may be necessary to protect the community and deny the criminal the opportunity to commit further crime, but punishment is merely cruelty. Some would argue that punishment may be justified because of its deterrent effect on others who might be thinking of committing similar crimes. The ethics of this reason for punishment – to discourage others – is, I think, very dubious.

On the other hand the deterministic viewpoint suggests the need to pick up early those at risk of behaving anti-socially, if possible before they have committed any crime. Treatment, if any is available, would, of course, be justified at this early stage. Whether detention at this stage is justified – for example of a man who has a strong propensity to assault and murder children – is difficult. However, if the risk of such criminal behaviour can be shown to be a high one I would argue in favour of offering such men the choice of either custodial care or regular medical treatment to reduce their sexual drive.

I do, of course, realise that in the first part of this discussion I was talking about the responsibility of parents in deciding how many children they will have, and in the second part I have suggested that we have little responsibility for our behaviour. The inconsistency is perhaps more apparent than real. Most of us are fortunate enough by, say, the age of twenty to develop personalities, predetermined perhaps, to allow us to make rational decisions based on the expected consequences of our actions. Most of us, too, have developed personalities such that we evaluate the probable consequences of our behaviour in part at least according to their effects on our fellow human beings including those of the next generation.

WILLIAMS I will follow Dr Carter in distinguishing two aspects of this subject: first, the question of our responsibility via genetic methods for the future, and, second, the influence of genetic determination on our ideas of individual responsibility. Unlike him I am going to, as it were, put the weight the other way round and say very little about the first and quite a bit more about the second.

About the first topic, namely our responsibility for the future by genetic means, I very largely agree with Dr Carter. I think that here, though, we do have to use a distinction which is an important, even if an unclear one, namely the distinction between trying to avoid gross evils on the one hand and trying to introduce improvement on the other. It seems to me that, particularly on the sort of liberal basis Dr Carter was for the most part taking for granted, we might very reasonably seek to avoid certain gross evils in the future by giving people advice with regard to the genetic consequences of the production of certain kinds of offspring. That would seem to be a perfectly rational and humane extension of our prudent social thoughts for the future.

What I find a great deal less appealing is the notion that was once popular, what used to be called Eugenics, the idea of improving the race by selective breeding. There seem to be at least two sorts of objection to this. One, which I won't labour, is the very evident incursions into freedom. The second difficulty is about the basis of values on which these supposed improvements would be introduced. One would have to take the kind of standpoint in which one regarded as self-evident to oneself what the future of the human race should be, presuppose that you knew what the human race was here for, and take all the steps you could to make it reach that ideal goal. But it is not at all clear where one is supposed to get that knowledge or information from. That is all I want to say about our responsibilities for the future race, and to say that I agree entirely with Carter about possible methods in which it could be brought to the attention of parents.

I want to turn now to the other subject, the relation of possible genetic determination to our views about people's responsibility for their actions. I think that genetic determination of people's motivation, behaviour and character, actually raises exactly the same issues of principle with regard to free will and responsibility as does any other form of determination and as are raised by any other form of scientific inquiry that bears on character, personality, and behaviour. Thus if we were given a set of scientific considerations drawn for instance from social psychology, or from psychoanalysis, or from certain kinds of sociology, which tended to show that people's character, motivation and behaviour patterns were determined, for instance, by the way they had been brought up or by certain formative features in their very early parental surroundings, or again by certain kinds of social conditions, were we given this information and the theory to go with it, then we would be faced with exactly the same problems with regard to individual responsibility, and freedom of the will, as we would be if given information to the effect that character was determined genetically.

But it might be said that, with regard to possible genetic determinations of character and behaviour, we are confronted with the problem in a somewhat more drastic form. The principal reason for this is that out of the sciences I have mentioned, it might seem that only a determination at a genetic level was likely to be represented in a scientific form sufficiently tough to count as, in fact, genuine determinism. It would seem very improbable that psychoanalysis, or considerations of sociology, are likely to produce other than general tendencies, or statistical propositions of some kind, which are unlikely to rise to the level of anything one would want really to call determinism; whereas it might be that genetic considerations in the context of a much expanded physiological understanding of the mind, an understanding of the mind at the level of the brain (here one is speculatively looking forward to very large developments in science) would give us an understanding, at a very tough level, of the determination of certain kinds of behaviour.

I suggest that it is unlikely that very highly determinate conditions of character and motivation will in general be discovered at the genetic level. My reason for thinking this is that we all know already that the influence of environmental considerations is extremely high in eliciting various kinds of social behaviour, character and motivation. What we might look for perhaps, in the understanding at genetic level, is certain kinds of potentialities, whether they be positive or negative, towards certain kinds of character, and these potentialities might be selectively developed or frustrated by certain kinds of environmental factors. I think I am right in claiming that we know this to be true, even with regard to physical characteristics; that is to say, you cannot say that a man's height is genetically determined, although you could say that the difference between two men's heights was genetically determined if they were brought up in the same environment.

This *a fortiore* is going to be true about behaviour, and I should like to draw attention to four respects which are important in limiting our ideas about the genetic determination of behaviour. The first is that some deviant or anti-social behaviour does not even represent any form of psychological abnormality. It just represents growing up normally in the deviant sub-group, as sociologists insist on calling it. That is, suppose, to take the simplest and crudest case, my parents are professional criminals and their friends are professional criminals, and the group in which I grow up is that of professional criminals, then I should be perfectly well-adjusted and genetically perfectly straightforward and come out a professional criminal. So that is at least one case in which deviance or, from the point of view of society, anti-social behaviour, would not represent any form of genetic peculiarity. Secondly, we have to remember the influence of what might be called luck. One form of luck turns up in a psychoanalytical consideration. For instance, it might well be the case that somebody has a kind of weakness, which would only be revealed by certain sorts of traumatic situations which with luck might be avoided. Thirdly, it may be, in a rather broader sense of luck, a matter of luck how certain sorts of character and drive, for instance of the destructive or irresponsible kind, find expression. That this is something which may be determined by social and family considerations is, I think, undeniable on grounds of common social observation. For instance, Dr Carter mentioned the very interesting case of men with XYY chromosomes, of whom a larger proportion than of other groups are found to end up as psychopathic characters. I don't think it is asserted, in fact I'm sure it is denied, that every person who has such a chromosomal defect will end up as a criminal. So this already suggests that although there's a greater probability or tendency in that direction, there are social and environmental factors at work which will tend to move somebody one way rather than another. Just from common observation, it is well known that there are certain patterns of drive, which might issue in behaviour which would land you in the criminal courts differentially depending upon what class you come from. For instance, if you come from working-class surroundings, having a character of this kind probably will end you up in the court. On the other hand, in better-favoured classes, it doesn't necessarily do so: you are merely the younger son who gets sent off into the army, or who used to be sent off into darkest Africa with a rifle but is now sent with a camera. Thus there is here a serious point about what form of expression destructive or irresponsible tendencies receive, and it is clear that something that may have a similar genetic basis in the case of two individuals, may, in fact, receive different expressions, some more overtly or notoriously anti-social than others, depending upon social and personal environmental circumstances, and features of luck.

Lastly, there is a general difficulty, in practice and theoretically, in determining what you regard as the boundaries of the genetic. There are, for instance, certain characteristics that can arise for genetic reasons. There is – and here I am walking into Dr Carter's territory – a condition known as phenylketonuria where, owing to a genetic deficiency, if the infant is given a standard diet the brain will degenerate and the child will turn into an idiot. If, however, this condition is detected early enough and the child is given a diet free of certain substances, degeneration will be avoided. This is a very interesting case, because in one sense the condition could be said to be genetically determined. On the other hand, selective interference with the environment will prevent the disability arising. Are you in this case to say that it is a genetically determined or an environmentally determined condition? Roughly, it is a genetically determined condition if you leave the environment normal; it is one of the classic cases, in which you do not properly know whether to call it genetic or not.

Suppose then we were convinced about the extent to which these various factors, not in the individual's own control, affected his character and motivation? How far would this affect our views about responsibility? This has been a subject for discussion by philosophers for a very long time and still is. It is one of the areas in philosophy in which some progress has been made. But despite that we do not know exactly how much of our moral vocabulary of right and wrong, 'responsibility', 'he could if he tried', 'he ought to have', 'he ought not to have', would survive what degree of scientific discovery about the formation of personality, and only to a certain extent can we determine this in advance by philosophical argument. To some extent we shall have to wait and see, but I think we can say one or two things *a priori*. People ask: 'Will there be a will if we discover that human character and motivation is, to a degree greater than at the moment we assume, determined by heredity and environment? Well, as a well-known philosopher used to say and quite properly, 'It all depends on what you mean by the will.' People have a concept of the will, which one might call the public school conception of the will, in which it is particularly associated with a characteristic called 'strength of will'. This is itself an ambiguous term. Strength of will is sometimes just sheer bloody-mindedness and in the extreme, has a psychopathic character, which we don't in fact wish to encourage. It also means: what makes people do things under difficult circumstances; sticking to it when the going gets hard; being prepared to jump into cold baths more rapidly than other people, and so forth. In that sense will is chiefly manifested by people who are, in fact, reluctant to do things. The man who needs a lot of will to be generous to other people is a person who does not particularly like being generous to other people. That consideration should make us sceptical, as it made the philosopher Hume sceptical, whether will is the central motion of morality, because it is unclear whether the central motion of morality has to be a characteristic which you only need if you really do not like doing the good thing.

In so far as strength of will in that sense is making yourself do things you do not like and is a characteristic that some people manifest more than others, it is just as likely to be determined by heredity and environment as anything else. So I would not put a lot of weight on will in that sense, as something which is going to prove immune to the advance of science and the understanding of character.

However, people sometimes mean by the will just ability to choose things. To me it seems that something like the ability to choose things must be compatible with any amount of determinism, if determinism is going to turn out to be true, for the very simple reason that choosing things is something we obviously do. If determinism is true at all, it's true now, obviously enough, though we don't know it is true yet. Hence anything that exists now is compatible with it, if it is true at all. But is it beyond question that, as things are, we choose? Well, let us say we do something very like it. Perhaps in some ultimate metaphysical sense, it might be argued that we don't choose now – it may be that we have a very exaggerated idea of how dignified and ultimate our choices are. But something goes on which, let us say, it is very easy to mistake for choosing, and very difficult to see why that should stop the day we discover determinism to be true.

There can be a concept of choice in which somebody only really chooses, decides, if he is not ultimately caused. In that sense it might be construed that we do not actually choose. But we certainly do something which is sufficiently like choosing for us to use that term and that's not going suddenly to stop because determinism turns out to be the case. The question is how important is this something like choice, that we have, going to prove when our scientific knowledge of character unrolls itself. I am now going to suggest two spheres relevant for our interpretation of our increasing scientific knowledge of the determination of character by genetics and environment.

First, we can distinguish between certain political and social set-ups which allow, in the political and social sense 'freedom of choice', and situations which do not allow that, and that distinction will still be valid even if determinism turns out to be true, because the difference between being hauled off, put in a van and told to do this, or being injected, or being brainwashed, and, on the other hand, having a chance to develop our own future, that distinction is going to survive, because there's still going to be a difference between subjugation and a degree of social and political freedom, even if everything about our characters is in general determined by heredity and environment. Because there is an obvious distinction between those two things – being kicked around by the management and not being kicked around by the management but given a bit of elbow room. And if determinism is true, it is true now, so this distinction is compatible with derminism being true now and will still be important, even if we find determinism to be true. That seems to me to give a very good reason for saying that the legal notion of the voluntary, the legal notion of responsibility – that is the motion that on the whole the State should not do nasty things to people unless those people have done anti-social things when roughly they knew what they were doing – that distinction will still be relevant, even though we learn a great deal more about determination of character by heredity and environment than we know at the moment. It will still be important to distinguish between the voluntary and the non-voluntary in the legal sense, and you do not have to believe in a metaphysical immaterial soul in order to uphold the distinction between the voluntary and the involuntary in a relevant sense, nor to uphold the values of justice.

Many people say these notions of responsibility are metaphysical nonsense, because things are actually determined by heredity and environment. So what we ought to do is turn over to social medicine and in particular, to preventive social medicine. One reason sometimes advanced for this is that it is unfair to punish criminals if in fact they are not, for reasons of heredity and environment, responsible for their actions, and therefore we ought to stop doing that and go in for social preventive medicine. The thing we have to remember here is that it does not make an awful lot of difference to how unpleasant it is being locked up, whether it is called punishment or it is called treatment. It does not make an awful lot of difference whether what is written on the front is H.M. Prison or H.M. Social Medical Prevention Centre, or whether it is run by the Home Office or the Ministry of Health. In both cases, the State is interfering with somebody and is taking them away and doing something to them. When it is said, 'It is unfair to punish criminals if their behaviour is the product of heredity and environment', this is a very weak line to take because the notion of unfairness being employed there is based on a set of values about justice with regard to which it must be at least as unfair to take away and put into a hospital somebody who has not done anything at all, but with regard to whom you have some apprehension that they might. To me it seems that either you believe in justice or you don't. If you believe in justice, then the proposed course is at least as nasty as the one that is being attacked and if you do not believe in justice, you cannot attack the prison practices for being unfair. What you can, of course, attack them for is not being effective. But then the question arises – effective for what? Just effectiveness to produce the maximum degree of social order? In that case, we would be back to injecting everybody in order to produce the maximum degree of quietness and conformity. There are, after all, other values beside social order and conformity, and one of them is justice.

I thought Dr Carter raised a question in this area when he asked: Are we punishing people because of deterrence? The ethics of deterrence is very problematical, if viewed from a basis of justice – that is, that you punish one sort of person in order to prevent certain conduct by others and this is unfair. But, again, we go through the same argument, namely that if unfairness is what we are at, then social preventive medicine must be at least as unfair as anything we do now. I don't believe that the increase of knowledge about the formation of character by heredity and environment is in principle going totally to sweep away the notions of the voluntary and the responsible, the notions of fairness and justice, and replace them by ideas of social preventive medicine.

The second point I want to make is that there is something very odd about the advocacy of replacing questions of the voluntary and justice, and so on, with questions of social preventive medicine by those theorists who say that the discovery of deterministic science of human behaviour is going to show that we can't choose anything. Because if it is going to show that we cannot choose anything, how can we choose these policies, namely, those of treating everybody one way, rather than another? If we can choose social policies, then we can choose a hell of a lot of other things besides, and so the notion of choice is not undermined. If we cannot choose even these policies, then it is very odd to go around producing a lot of rational reasons to try and persuade us to adopt them.

The Chairman then invited questions from the audience.

G. S. ERWIN Dr Carter, is the fear of bearing a deformed child ever strong enough to cause total avoidance of maternity?

CARTER The short answer is yes, certainly. I know very many parents who have had a handicapped child and are so afraid of having another, that they have decided to have no more children and have adopted instead. It is a common situation, and one of our jobs in genetic clinics is to make sure that they get good advice before they decide one way or the other, because all too often their fears are unjustified.

MISS B. HODGEKINSON Has Dr Carter any positive evidence that the gene mutation rate is influenced strongly by radiation?

CARTER It has been very clearly shown that the mutation rate can be increased by ionising radiation. What we do not know at all accurately in humans is the size of the effect, but again we are getting some fairly good indications of what the limitations are. A good example is from the excellent follow-up study that has been done in Hiroshima and Nagasaki of those exposed to radiation from the first two atomic bombs, and I think it is right to say that no concrete demonstration has come from this survey of any increase in mutation rate. This sets us some limit to the size of the effect but that there is some effect is not in doubt and also there is no safe dosage; even a small dose of radiation will have a tiny effect.

E. HERSHON I should like to ask Dr Carter whether there is any danger to our future genetic health in modern medicine, making such conditions as cleft palate and phenylketonuria viable, whereas they would normally be weeded out by natural selection?

CARTER If no counter measures were taken, then one would expect a small steady slow increase in the proportion of children born with these conditions. The way round this dilemma is, of course, genetic counselling. If you tell parents what the risks are so that they, some of them at least, plan a family size below replacement rate, you prevent this increase. In fact, with genetic counselling you can do very much better than natural selection. You can move much faster, so we are not worried about this problem, provided we do our bit about genetic counselling. Take phenylketonuria, for example; you cannot have children with this condition unless two carriers of the gene marry each other. The solution to that in the long run is to find out, perhaps as part of the school medical service, who are carriers, then warn them against marrying each other. If they insist on marrying each other, you may before long be able to pick up the child who is going to be phenylketonuric early in the pregnancy and offer the mother a termination. Whether that should be done when we have a good treatment – not a hundred per cent treatment, though pretty effective – is an ethical problem which the parents would have to decide on in consultation with their doctors.

MARION WALKER Would Dr Carter advise that any parents of a Mongol child should have tests to see whether there is a one-in-four chance of recurrence or whether it is purely accidental?

CARTER Yes, certainly, if the mother is under the age of thirty when she has a Mongol baby, and she is thinking about having further children, we would recommend that she gets advice and this will almost certainly involve chromosome tests, at least on the baby, if not on both parents. If she is over thirty, it is so likely to be of the accidental type that while our laboratory facilities are in short supply, we would rather not do the test because the chance of it being positive is small. But when the mother is under thirty, it is well worth picking up the five per cent with a high risk. And, looking a little to the future, even if there is a high risk, if the mother is prepared to take it, we may be able to see if she has been unlucky early in the pregnancy and offer her a termination if she has.

A. N. OTHER If there came a time when we could determine that, say, an individual is likely to produce offspring who are either dangerous to society or parasitic upon society, what are the ethics of interfering by sterilisation of that individual?

WILLIAMS If you are asking what I personally think of the idea, I think very poorly of it and am against it, and think it would be wrong. If it's a question about what principles are involved in giving such an answer, my answer would be as follows. The question is, has the State the right to interfere with something which is of great intimacy, privacy, and personal choice? To justify interference on the basis of a possible hazard of very generally defined disadvantages would be very difficult indeed. In general, gross restrictions on individual choices have to be justified on the grounds of something that they have done, or a clear and present danger of some very large-scale result that might follow. I am putting this in very utilitarian terms, but that seems to me the rights and wrongs of it, and I think it very unlikely that we will come anywhere near such a condition in practical terms.

CARTER I would agree with that. I think, in practice, the question hardly ever arises. If you have a man or a woman who has a high risk of having a severely mentally retarded child for genetic reasons, all you have to do is to explain the risk and provide them with the opportunity for family planning. Some of them may ask for sterilisation and if that is the best solution and that is what they want, one is prepared to help them, but compulsory sterilisation is not a practical issue and is not necessary.

B. MINTY A question for Professor Williams. Apropos your remark about there not being much difference in practice between Her Majesty's social preventive centre and Her Majesty's prison, would you say that the discovery that certain kinds of behaviour is due to sickness rather than to wickedness has not helped us at all? That this has not been insight?

WILLIAMS Well, of course it has been an insight. What is it that was believed when it was believed to be due to wickedness? If it consisted of the belief that if you address the man sternly enough and offered him sufficient moral condemnation, then it is only pure bloody-mindedness on his part if he then does not choose to toe the line: that is, he always could have toed the line had he wished to. Well, obviously, that belief is in many cases false. In a large number of cases, it is obviously enlightening, just to stop people persecuting others in a particularly reprobatory kind of way, whereas otherwise they might have done this. This is absolutely true. You also stop believing something which is untrue, which is always an advantage. I think it may further be the case that people in the past who were recidivists because of various psychological conditions, were subjected to cruel and inhumane punishments because of people's false beliefs about them. If these beliefs are suspended, so much the better. But if the only difference between the social preventive centre and the prison is that the man is incarcerated under rather more agreeable conditions, that is an improvement, though not one which makes the ends different to a man who would like to regard himself as perfectly free. I would agree that there are advances associated with the distinction between sickness and wickedness, though the distinction is not always as clear as it might be.

CARTER I might add one point there. I think one of the distinctions is that if you look on certain types of criminal behaviour as sickness and you provide a treatment, then detention is going to be very short. There is no question of sentence for five years or ten years. And so this view of crime as sickness works both ways. You may find that somebody has to be in preventive detention for life. You may also in many instances find they can be let out in a fortnight providing they respond to the necessary treatment.

WILLIAMS I think that many issues come into this one. It is a very large issue, as everybody knows. I think that, as Professor Hart and others have said, one of the issues that has to be borne in mind from the preventive point of view, is that it is a value of the law, that ought to be preserved as far as possible, that you can know in advance what you are likely to get caught for; that is, the old provisions against retrospective offences, and that the law should be fairly stable and fairly predictable within admittedly extremely imperfect limits. All these factors are connected with provisions of justice, which mean that a man can arrange his life within the limits of the law, if he so chooses. If somebody suddenly looks as if he's getting a bit sickly, and he's beginning to put out spots in the direction of anti-social behaviour he may find himself subject to interference by the State in a way not predictable by him – this really does offend against certain values.

COHEN But he may find himself restricted in a predictable way. If he has an infectious disease, and there is the likelihood that the community in which he lives may be at risk, the law does say he must not expose the community to that risk. Is there any great difference between that and the man whose social illness exposes the community in which he lives to certain dangers and so therefore he is detained because of that?

WILLIAMS Yes, quite a number of differences. One is that infectious illnesses are fundamentally concerned with things that happen to him and not things that he does, and hence his infectious illness is by himself seen as a limitation on his freedom of action. If I get measles this is for me a limitation on what I want to do, whereas if I engage in illegal activities, these activities are not limitations on what I want to do – they are precisely what I want to do. Hence there is an identification with my projects which make them a part of me in a way in which there isn't an identification with my diseases which would make them part of me. Hence the restrictions on these activities are restrictions in quite a different sense.

COHEN If a person is socially ill and his illness takes the form of molesting or killing young girls, I would have thought that there might be reason for regarding that as in a similar way a community danger.

WILLIAMS Well of course he has to be restrained if he's going to go around molesting or killing small girls. This is obviously true. In such a case what we would recognise as gross psychopathic illness, psychological illness, these medical categories would no doubt come in. But there is a difference. What about a man who just likes, or is concerned with, certain deviant behaviour such as stealing. Now he himself recognises, in the case of an infectious disease, that this is a misfortune for him which, other things being equal, he would not wish to give to others, but the man who has these deviant policies does not regard them like a misfortune for him. He may see it as a misfortune for other people but it really doesn't make much difference in what ways and to what depths you are affecting his freedom, and very often we use the expression 'social sickness' because we think that more is justified in the name of medicine than would be justified in the name of the law.

KELLY I am a little worried about Professor Williams's position on the question of moral responsibility. He is prepared, apparently, to regard certain types of people, such as XYY psychopaths, as being morally irresponsible, but seems also to have a concept of a normal human being who is morally responsible in spite of everything that the psychologists and the sociologists can do to us. I wonder what really a normal human being is, and whether in fact we are faced with, not a difference between responsibility and irresponsibility, but a sliding scale of responsibility.

WILLIAMS I don't think I ever said anything else. I wasn't aware of using the categories 'morally responsible' and 'not responsible' in this very open and shut way. I quite agree with you. I think that the point is this. If you take the various legal categories we employ, then these have an appearance, probably an accepted appearance, of being open and shut categories. As the lawyer sometimes put it; did he have a guilty mind or not? But so often in the law, the open and shut case appearance of it is in fact a formulation for a set of more or less balanced and weighed considerations, and it is in this light that people actually have to assess these cases. What I was really talking about was somebody who takes a very drastic view and says, 'Well, actually nobody's morally responsible for anything.' It is sometimes suggested that if we really believed in determinism we could not think of people making choices at all. To me, that is a very unrealistic position. We would certainly have to use sliding scales, of people being more or less responsible for various things under different circumstances, and there is also the question of there being more than one scale.

For instance, we have three central questions related to responsibility, both in law and everyday life. One is, Was it he that did it? Secondly, Did he mean to do it, or was he, for instance, ignorant of what he was doing? and thirdly, Could he help doing it? because it may be that he knew what it was, but he couldn't help doing it, or very often of course in everyday cases, he could have helped doing it in the ordinary sense, it wasn't that he had a compulsion to do it, but he didn't mean to do it – he really intended to do something else; he just pulled the wrong lever or something. There are these three dimensions at least. Who was it?, Did he mean it?, and Could he help it? – all of which have to be employed in assessing responsibility. The conditions of *determinism* are particularly connected with 'could he help it?', rather than 'did he mean it?' *Psycho-*

analytical explanations are really explanations that are more connected with, 'did he mean it?', than 'could he help it?'

COHEN One of the problems here is exemplified by the XYY chromosome. Let us suppose that the XYY has been identified as the cause of deviant behaviour. That's a comparatively recent discovery and indeed, until a few years ago, there would have been no means of discovering that particular physical abnormality. What would we have said about this deviant behaviour before we had determined that there was a physical basis to it?

WILLIAMS That is an extremely interesting historical question, which I think might well admit an historical answer. We probably overestimate the amount of time that past ages spent in moralistic rhetoric about what we recognise as pathological conditions, partly because all ages over-react to the last one, or the last but one. We have a particular view of some Victorian moralistic judge sounding off, or a Victorian parent. But that apart, past ages did have the notion that some people had unusually and dangerously violent temperaments; we have added further dimensions of explanation to that notion. And partly (though only partly) for that reason, we may hope to deal with such cases in less inhumane ways.

COHEN I think at this point I should attempt a brief summing up. Both our speakers were concerned with two main themes. Professor Williams emphasised the moral responsibility of the present generation for the genetic endowment of the next, and Dr Carter told us that the genetic constitutions of offspring cannot be determined with certainty, but that there are varying degrees of probability, as high as one in four in relation to certain diseases, such as types of deafness, or types of blindness, and the like, but others have a much lower degree of probability. And most of those that have a high degree of probability depend upon single gene inheritance rather than on many genes producing a particular phenotype as we call it: a particular individual characteristic rather than a genotype. Also, we are now able to determine in many instances that those who are not suffering from a disease may yet carry the gene which could convey the disease to their offspring. The methods of determining these have been increased in accuracy and delicacy in recent years. Dr Carter has said, and I think that Professor Williams agrees, that the decision as to whether to accept the risk is one for the parents and not for the community, though it is the community's duty to provide the means whereby accurate genetic counselling can be obtained by those who wish to have it, or, if an abnormality can be determined prenatally, that a parent should decide whether abortion should follow.

The second theme to which they devoted attention, this one rather more by Professor Williams, is how far does genetic constitution predetermine an individual's responsibility for his behaviour and thus limit his moral responsibility for it. In other words, in what degree have we free will? Dr Carter pointed out that certain people with psychotic disturbances, schizophrenia, and the like, had little or no responsibility for their behaviour, and he dealt with the chromosome abnormalities which are concerned. I thought that he perhaps tilted his views towards the determinist outlook more at any rate than did Professor Williams who rather said: 'Well, it depends on how you look at this, and even if there is a determined outlook we still have a choice.' It has occurred to me that it is perhaps a mistake to think of either the total picture as genetic determination or of environmental determination, and certainly in the psychological field to think in terms of one or other.

Throughout these discussions we have discussed the individual, social and ethical problems to which advances in medicine have given rise. We are grateful to all who have contributed to the discussions.